How to Fight FATflammation!

HOW TO FIGHT
FATflammation!

*A Revolutionary 3-Week Program
to Shrink the Body's Fat Cells
for Quick and Lasting Weight Loss*

Lori Shemek, Ph.D., CNC, CLC

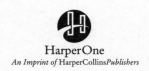

HarperOne
An Imprint of HarperCollinsPublishers

HarperOne

This book contains advice and information relating to health care. It should be used to supplement rather than replace the advice of your doctor or another trained health professional. If you know or suspect that you have a health problem, it is recommended that you seek your physician's advice before embarking on any medical program or treatment. All efforts have been made to ensure the accuracy of the information contained in this book as of the date of publication. The publisher and the author disclaim liability for any medical outcomes that may occur as a result of applying the methods suggested in this book.

FIRST EDITION

Designed by Terry McGrath

Library of Congress Cataloging-in-Publication Data
Shemek, Lori.
How to fight fatflammation! : a revolutionary 3-week program to shrink the body's fat cells for quick and lasting weight loss / Lori Shemek, Ph.D., CNC, CLC.
    pages cm
ISBN 978-0-06-234753-4
1. Reducing diets. 2. Weight loss. 3. Fat cells. 4. Inflammation. I. Title.
RM222.2.S5254 2015
613.2'5—dc23

                    2015001469

15 16 17 18 19   RRD(H)   10 9 8 7 6 5 4 3 2 1

To the memory of my beautiful mother, Sally Ann,
and all others who share her struggles with weight.

CONTENTS

Part Four

FATFLAMMATION FREE FOREVER!

Appendix

Allowed Foods and Recipes

INTRODUCTION

▶ I grew up with a single mother who didn't think she had many choices in life, nor did she believe she deserved health or happiness. Consequently, my sweet mother created a life that was a testament to poor decision making. She was, understandably, always stressed; we had little or no money; her personal life was a mess; she gravitated toward questionable relationships; she smoked heavily; she sometimes drank to excess and always ate badly, putting a personal emphasis on sugar. She was very overweight and suffered from a myriad of small and large health-related issues. Most of my memories of my mother involve watching her suffer from one physical problem after another.

Even as a child, I was interested in health and knew intuitively that my mother's choices were doing her in. I was always shocked that my mother, a trained nurse, took such poor care of herself, and I remember pleading with her to stop eating cookies and start taking vitamins. I also remember struggling to create a healthier lifestyle for myself and my two younger brothers, whose care was often left to me.

My mother died at thirty-six, just a week after I turned seventeen. My personal *aha!* moment came at her memorial service when I vividly remember saying to myself: *She didn't have to die. She could have made better decisions. She could have made different choices!* Right then, I decided what I wanted to do with my life: I wanted to help people make healthier choices.

With this in mind, I finished high school, and focused on finding a way to get to college. After earning a Ph.D. in psychology, I got a job as a casework therapist for a nonprofit organization in Dallas dedicated to the prevention of child abuse and neglect. But as committed as I was to the emotional well-being of our clients, I never let go of my interest in diet and health. When I visited our client families, I couldn't help but notice how poorly some of them were eating. I began creating nutritional plans for families that would include giving up sugar and soda and introducing fruit and vegetables, and when some of these mothers began following my advice, we could all see the improvements in their lives in very dramatic ways. My work allowed me to see firsthand the extent to which physical health seriously impacts emotional health and vice versa. In my off-hours, I also started creating nutritional plans for friends. It was becoming more and more apparent to me that I needed to find a way to fulfill my lifelong interest in diet and nutrition, so I left my job. My goal was to marry my background in psychology with my strong commitment to good health and nutrition. With that I mind, I earned my certification in nutritional counseling, and because I wanted to know more techniques and ways of helping people, I also became a certified life coach.

My personal dream is to help as many people as possible achieve more satisfying lives. I want to help people with weight issues create positive change and alter the way they view themselves in relation to the world. I want them to realize that they have greater control and always have the option of making different choices. My mission and passion is to help men and women who need to lose weight get to a weight where they not only feel healthy, but also have an improved sense of self-worth.

This is why I designed the FATflammation-Free Diet. I've had clients who have lost 20 pounds, and I've had clients who have lost 200 pounds. I know it can be done.

The FATflammation-Free Diet Program will change the way your fat cells operate. Your body will naturally and effortlessly be trained to stop your fat cells from overexpanding. As soon as you begin to reduce the inflammation within the cells, you will immediately reboot your body chemistry: your fat cells will become healthy again and shrink, and, as they do, unwanted pounds will melt away.

It's important for you to understand that it's more about *what you eat*, not how much you eat, that causes weight gain and FATflammation. Research shows there are specific foods that target inflamed, overstuffed fat cells. The FATflammation-Free Diet Program is going to teach you which foods you need to avoid and which foods are going to help you get thin.

So let's get started.

PART ONE

HOW FATFLAMMATION MAKES YOU FAT

CHAPTER 1

WHY CUTTING CALORIES DOESN'T CUT IT

▶ For years we have been told that a calorie is a calorie is a calorie. We've been told that a hundred calories of mixed green vegetables is exactly the same as one hundred calories of chocolate syrup. Anyone who has ever been on a diet has probably known intuitively that this is not the case. But that's what science was telling us. Now, though, science has finally acknowledged that there is a difference between the way the body metabolizes green vegetables and chocolate syrup. Like other sugars and refined carbohydrates, chocolate syrup makes blood sugar and insulin spike. This, in turn, causes fatter fat cells. When you put two teaspoons of sugar into your coffee or tea, you immediately set the process of FATflammation in motion. The nutrient-rich mixed green vegetables, on the other hand, will balance your blood sugar, help restore balance to the body, and reduce inflammation within your cells, thus fueling up your fat burn.

The old-fashioned way of dieting by cutting calories also doesn't work, because if you cut too many calories and eat too little food, your body senses it is lacking fuel and slows down your metabolism to conserve energy. Then, if you increase your calories and go back to your normal way of eating, your metabolism has become sluggish and thus you store fat.

Here's the first thing I want to tell anyone who is trying to lose weight: Forget everything you've ever been told. Forget about counting calories, counting points, weighing your food, fad diets, no-fat diets, or spending countless hours at the gym. There is a better way, a more reliable, and satisfying way to lose the fat and maintain your desired weight.

By now, we all know that the Standard American Diet (SAD), which typically includes fast food, isn't good for our health or our weight. But even men and women who have never set foot into a McDonald's or a Burger King have issues with their weight. That's because we have been misinformed about what we should and shouldn't eat to stay healthy and fit. Here's a secret: many of the foods we have been told are healthy are actually unhealthy and encourage inflammation. Some examples of this include fat-free foods, soy milk, yogurt with fruit, protein bars, and many of the most popular vegetable and seed oils that are used just about everywhere—from cooking oil to salad dressings like canola, corn, safflower, and soy.

WHEN FAILED DIETS HAPPEN TO GOOD PEOPLE

"I certainly understand how I got fat," Carrie told me when I first met her. "I wasn't careful about what I put in my mouth. What I don't understand is why I can't lose it. Sometimes it seems as though my fat has a life of its own."

I understood why Carrie, a forty-four-year-old veterinary tech, was feeling so frustrated. She had already been dieting off and on for more than a year and nothing she was doing was helping her win the weight war. "For years," she said, "I ate everything in sight without thinking about what it was doing to my body. But now even though I'm being supercareful, the weight doesn't go away."

Carrie, who is married and has a twelve-year-old daughter, gained weight the same way that many of us do. By not paying attention. "I would start every day making breakfast for my daughter, Jessie, and packing her lunch," she told me, describing her issues with fat and food. "While I did that I would sort of snack my way around the kitchen. If I made her pancakes or oatmeal, I would eat a little bit while I was cooking. I would also have my usual breakfast, which is juice, toast, and coffee. Every time I opened the refrigerator or a cabinet, I ate a bite of something—a little piece of cheese, half a slice of bread, a spoonful of peanut butter, a cookie, a handful of chips or raisins, some crackers. It was all just nervous, distracted eating. Whatever I ate, I did it standing up so it never felt like I was really having a meal. When I got to work, right away I would have another cup of coffee with a toasted bagel, buttered or with cream cheese. Sometimes I also had a yogurt."

"Plain yogurt or one with a little bit of fruit and lots of sugar?" I asked her.

"Fruit," she replied. "I always forget that yogurt has sugar. I like peach, but it was always low fat or no fat. Does it have much sugar?"

"At least fourteen grams or more per container, and usually more," I nodded. "That's like eating a donut."

For lunch, Carrie told me, she usually had soup and a sandwich and some kind of caffeinated diet soda. She loves chocolate, so in the middle of the afternoon, she sometimes had a hot chocolate or another diet soda.

As far as dinner was concerned, Carrie and her husband both work full days so they shared responsibility. "We're tired during the week so when I was putting on the weight, our meals were pretty much hit or miss. My husband would bring home a pizza or a barbecued chicken, or we would order in Chinese or Thai food. Our daughter is kind of picky. She sort of always wants to eat the same thing—chicken fingers or grilled cheese or pasta with meat sauce. Sometimes I would make something that we would all eat—like chicken parm with pasta.

"In the summer, my husband would grill hamburgers, steak, or barbecued chicken, and we'd have corn, salad or cold slaw. My biggest weakness is pasta so I would have chicken, steak, corn, and salad with my husband and pasta with my daughter. My husband loves sweets and he is always bringing home donuts, cookies, candy, and ice cream. Before I went to bed, I would eat a little bit of everything, including the ice cream, especially if it was chocolate. And I also never seemed to have time to exercise. Between work and being a mom, I just didn't have the time. That's how I put on the weight. It was easy.

"About a year and a half ago, I finally admitted that I had gained at least thirty-five to forty pounds—more weight than I was going to be able to lose by starving myself for a weekend. Nothing I own really fits me anymore. I'm five foot eight and have big bones so I can hide some weight on my frame. But even so, I was embarrassed to go anywhere, and I started wearing baggy jackets so nobody could see how fat I was. That's when I started to get serious about trying to lose weight. Now, I'm eating less than half as much food as I used to, but I'm barely maintaining. I think I've tried every diet, and maybe I lose a pound of two, but I can't keep it off. It seems to me that every week I am eating less and less food and having fewer and fewer calories. There are no more chips or cookies in my life, and I started exercising. My cousin gave me her 'barely used' exercise bike and I do use it—at least three or four times a week. I really need to do something about the cellulite. I want to be able to hang out at the pool without covering up. So I'm also trying to walk every afternoon at lunch. But, no matter what I do or how little I eat, I'm not losing weight. Why does this happen? Why didn't any of the diets I've been on work? Sometimes it seems as though my fat has a life of its own."

Well, guess what? Carrie's right. *Our fat cells do have a life of their own!*

Most diets fail because they don't get to the root of the problem—inflamed fat cells. Something that many of us have suspected for a long time turns out to be true. Science now tells us that our fat cells do have their very own agenda. Researchers have recently discovered a unique form of chronic inflammation that is taking place in the fat cells in our bodies. We now know that there is a real and workable solution to our issues with weight. If we want to fix our problems with fat, we need to reduce the inflammation in our fat cells.

Let's start out by saying that we all have fat cells. Thin people have fat cells. Children have fat cells. And, yes, people with weight problems have fat cells. On its own, this isn't a problem. Your fat cells have a primary function, which is to act as a storage unit. Your fat cells hold the energy you get from the food you eat. Soon after you eat, your fat cells enlarge to hold all the free fatty acids and glucose contained in your breakfast, lunch, dinner, or snack. The energy found in the food is then sent out as fuel to feed the various parts of your body as needed. A healthy fat cell is incredibly small—a very small fraction of the size of the period at the end of this sentence—and it functions optimally at that size. Like an accordion, it swells up after you eat, and then goes back to its ideal size after it has finished its job. But many of us no longer have fat cells that function like this. Instead our fat cells have become inflamed, bloated, and swollen. That's why we get fat, and this is a fixable problem—and it can be done quickly.

QUESTION: **What causes the fat cells in our body to become inflamed?**
ANSWER: **Wrong food choices = Inflamed fat cells = Weight gain**

Here is the big problem: many of the foods we all eat as part of our regular diet irritate our fat cells, causing them to become chronically oversized and inflamed. They swell up, but they don't go down. As fat cells get swollen and inflamed, an inflammatory cycle is put in motion. This silent, insidious process is what makes us fat.

Because this chronic weight-inducing inflammation is caused and controlled by the foods we eat—some foods are inflammatory; some are anti-inflammatory—we can fix our problems with fat! The FATflammation-Free Diet Program tells you which foods to eat and which ones to avoid to permanently and speedily shrink your fat cells.

INFLAMMATION AND FAT

In the last few years, inflammation has become one of the most talked about subjects in medicine. That's because researchers have become acutely aware of the role inflammation plays in the development of disease—heart disease, Alzheimer's, arthritis, strokes, diabetes, and even depression, just to name a few. What they are only now beginning to discuss is the key, though often overlooked role inflammation plays in weight gain. That's why I call it FAT-flammation™.

Let's start by talking more about what inflammation is and how it reveals itself in our bodies. For a moment, think about the kind of thing that happened to most of us when we were kids. Do you remember falling off your bicycle or your skates and skinning your knee? Remember how your knee looked after you hurt yourself? Perhaps it was black and blue and bruised. Perhaps you scraped your skin and it all turned red and disgusting looking. Perhaps you cut yourself, falling on a dirty sidewalk, and the cut became infected. In short, when you looked at your knee in the day or so after your little accident, you could clearly see the inflammation. This is what acute inflammation looks like.

What we know then is that inflammation is a natural reaction that takes place in body in response to injury, infection, or the introduction of a foreign substance that is toxic or allergy producing. Acute inflammation, which usually lasts a short time, is a necessary part of the healing process.

Therefore, after that unfortunate bike accident, your knee probably cleared up within a week or so, and the inflammation went away. But let's suppose that you did what you were told not to do—you picked at the scab that formed on your knee, or you weren't careful and you fell again, thus reinjuring your knee in the same place. Instead of healing, what happened then is that the inflammation stayed with you, and it became chronic.

I can hear your next question: "So what does this have to do with my gaining weight?"

Here's your answer: the foods you choose to eat are irritating and reirritating your fat cells. Even some so-called healthy foods are actually injuring them, causing them to become chronically inflamed. And inflamed fat cells are what make you fat. You may be choosing to eat the same kind of foods every day; in this way your fat cells are continually under assault.

In short, the same kind of inflammatory response that took place in your knee, when you injured it and then reinjured it, can take place in each and every one of your fat cells, particularly those in your abdominal area. Think of a chronically irritated fat cell as being like a small factory churning out inflammatory molecules. When this happens, your metabolism responds by slowing down. A slower metabolism leads to more weight gain, which, in turn, results in more inflammation. This sets up a vicious cycle, because when your fat cells are irritated or inflamed, they release even more inflammatory molecules.

The more weight you gain, the greater the inflammation, which leads to more weight gain. Infections, as we know, cause inflammation. Weight gain actually makes your fat cells behave as though they are infected. When the fat cells in your body are regularly inflamed, the situation becomes chronic. This is FATflammation.

LOSING *YOUR* FAT—WHAT YOU NEED TO DO

Here's the good news: if an inflammatory diet can cause FATflammation, an anti-inflammatory diet that targets fat cells directly can reverse the process. The newest research on diet and health is breathtakingly clear on the role of inflammation and fat. The minute you give up the foods that cause inflammation and increase your dietary intake of foods that fight inflammation, you will start to fix your problems with fat. The FATflammation-Free Diet Program will provide a wide range of healthy as well as delicious food choices to help you change the way you eat.

What Causes FATflammation?

Dehydration
Sugar and artificial sweeteners
High-fructose corn syrup
Trans fats
Refined grains
Foods high in omega-6 oils, such as corn, peanut, soybean, safflower, and sunflower oil
Imbalanced digestive bacteria
Foods to which you are allergic or have a specific sensitivity
Stress
A lack of sleep
Too little exercise

What Fights FATflammation?

Water

Protein

Cultured foods and probiotics

**Omega-3 fatty acids (found in cold water fish and Omega-3
   supplements)**

Healthy oils such as coconut oil, olive oil, and macadamia nut oil

Fiber

Micronutrients (minerals, vitamins, and phytonutrients)

Eliminating foods to which you might be allergic or sensitive

Mindfulness

Sleep

Regular exercise

Change your dietary habits and your fat cells respond by going down in size. I know this because I have seen it happen. The FATflammation-Free Diet Program is a science-based approach to weight loss that will absolutely help anyone with weight issues become leaner, thinner, and more energized as well as happier and healthier.

THE WOMAN WHO ATE NEXT TO NOTHING

I will always remember Lorna, whose inability to lose weight was making her feel, as she put it, as though she was "at the end of her rope." Lorna, an outgoing woman with an upbeat personality, an active life, and a great spirit, also loved to cook. To cut calories, however, she had stopped cooking and was relying mostly on prepared and take-out food. Lorna realized that she needed to lose about forty pounds, but it wasn't coming off. She was as perplexed as she was frustrated. I could understand her frustration and unhappiness because she really was eating very little. But her food choices were unknowingly making her bloated and tired as well as perpetually fat.

Each morning Lorna would start the day with coffee and a roll on which she put a little bit of butter substitute. For lunch, she would go to a local restaurant and take out a roast beef sandwich on a roll made from refined grains, as well as a salad. She loved the little packages of dressing that came with the salad so she would often ask for two, which she would put on her salad. Sometimes she took a third package of dressing to have at home. At night she would have some kind of frozen dinner—often fried chicken. If she made herself a salad at home, which she sometimes did, she used one of those extra packages of dressing. She typically also had several diet sodas during the day.

Lorna told me that she often felt hungry, but her desire to lose weight kept her determined, and she stuck with her reduced-calorie diet. I don't know how she did it. She was a prime example of someone who was overweight as well as malnourished and deficient in vitamins, minerals, and other essential nutrients. It was a tribute to her great life force and spirit that she didn't get discouraged and give up.

It was easy to get a handle on why Lorna's "diet" wasn't helping her get rid of her fat. Almost everything she ate was inflammatory. Her breakfast was inflammatory because the roll was made with refined grains and she used a butter substitute that included inflammatory omega-6 oils. The roast beef in her sandwich was okay, but she was eating it on another roll made from inflammatory refined grains. The salad was good, but the dressing contained inflammatory omega-6 oils and highly inflammatory high-fructose corn syrup (HFCS). The chicken in her frozen dinner was coated with an inflammatory refined grain and fried in inflammatory omega-6 oil. And each time Lorna took a sip of her diet soda, she was adding more inflammation to her life in the form of artificial sweeteners.

Helping Lorna lose her fat wasn't complicated. I suggested that she immediately begin taking a daily supplement that included 4,000 mg of omega-3 fish oil. We also immediately removed all the omega-6 oils in her diet and replaced them with healthy omega-3 fats and oils—olive oil, macadamia nut oil, coconut oil, avocados, olives, nuts, and nut butters—that are able to reverse FATflammation. She stopped eating refined grains like white bread, and she began eating small amounts of grains like quinoa and brown rice. She ate more complex carbohydrates in the form of nonstarchy green vegetables, such as broccoli, spinach, kale, asparagus, and string beans. I also told Lorna that she needed to include more protein, particularly omega-3 rich fish such as salmon.

Because Lorna needed to eat more food, not less, and more frequently throughout the day, I asked her to change her diet so that she was having three meals a day and two snacks, and I told her to include protein with every meal and snack. From what Lorna told me about her fluid intake, it was apparent that she was also dehydrated. Because water is a powerful inflammation fighter, I told her to start drinking more water. I also suggested that she take a probiotic supplement, which became part of her daily routine. Lorna started getting rid of her fat almost immediately. She lost eight pounds in her first week and her bloated belly shrunk two inches. By staying on the FATflammation-Free Diet Program, she fixed her problems with fat. You can do the same.

DON'T BE EMBARRASSED AND DON'T BLAME YOURSELF

When we gain weight, we often become embarrassed about how we look. We tend to enter into a world of self-blame. *How did I let this happen?* is a typical question we ask ourselves. We start to avoid full-length mirrors. Even walking past our reflection in a glass store window can be traumatic. We look at the reflection and wonder, *Who is that flabby fat person staring back at me? That can't be me!* Fat makes us feel upset and ashamed. It makes us hide our weight behind oversized jackets and large shirts. It makes us reluctant to attend family events and class reunions. It makes us avoid going on first dates with strangers. We wonder things like, *What will he/she think of me?* It can sometimes even make us embarrassed in front of our significant others, not to mention our own children (particularly if they are adolescents). Unfortunately, these reactions tend to make us want to hide out and retreat further into our own comfort zone, which, understandably, is frequently in front of the TV with a bag of chips or a handful of M&Ms.

Carrying around too much fat is an emotional burden as well as a physical one. I don't know anybody who started out saying, "I want to be overweight! Bring on the fat!" Nonetheless, just about all the people I've counseled with weight issues tend to blame themselves. I want to start by telling you that there are dozens of reasons why any one of us might pack on the pounds and get "overfat." Some of reasons are metabolic; some are genetic—these can both be dealt with. But let's not forget a major reason why we put on weight: even though we have more food choices than ever before, poor and inflammatory food choices are everywhere and vastly outnumber the good. In fact, many of the foods we've been encouraged to eat, such as soy milk and low-fat dairy products, can fuel FATflammation.

I'm not saying that the food industry prioritized creating foods that would make us fat and unhealthy. I'm not even accusing the food industry of planning to give us more cellulite. I'm sure it's all been inadvertent. Nonetheless, that's what has happened. Anyone who has ever been stuck waiting for a train, bus, or plane knows what it's like to try to find a healthy food option. Just about everything available is unhealthy, fattening, and inflammatory. Bus and train stations specialize in donut franchises and vending machines that contain nothing but cookies, chips, and candy. And, if you decide to opt for a little package of peanut butter crackers, thinking *How "fattening" could this be?*, take a look at the inflammatory ingredients listed on the labels. The choices at airports are only marginally better. Perhaps you can find flavored yogurt or little containers of fruit salad, but both are loaded with added sugar, a major cause of inflammation. It's even amazingly difficult to find a sandwich that hasn't been made with questionable ingredients. But these choices are not limited to facilities where we are forced to rely on what we can get from machines or vendors selling prepared foods.

Our own kitchens have become danger zones. For example, take a look at the ingredients in some of the soups produced by well-known American companies. The happy little cans visually appear to be almost the same as they were in Grandma's day. Didn't many of us grow up loving canned tomato soup in Mom's or Grandma's kitchen? The problem is that the soup we are eating today is no longer the same product it was twenty or thirty years ago. It is now laden with ingredients that have little to do with anything that was created naturally. Round up the usual suspects—too much sodium, sugar, and high-fructose corn syrup, all of which are highly inflammatory. And, for whatever it's worth, many of these canned soups also have more calories than they did in Grandma's day.

Here's a good question to ask: Why is sugar or HFCS in our soup? Here's the answer: food manufacturers, who want to sell their products, know that people are addicted to the sweet stuff. High-fructose corn syrup is less expensive than sugar; that's why many manufacturers started using it instead of sugar. Now it seems as though it is in everything. These days, it is challenging to find food that isn't in some way adding to our problem with fat, but, I want to assure you, that it can be done, which is one of the reasons why I created the FATflammation-Free Diet Program.

Another major problem: the food and medical experts have also given us the wrong advice, all of which has contributed to our problems with weight. For years we were told to avoid anything with fat and instead choose foods that are primarily carbohydrate. We now know that this advice has added to our problems and made us fat. That's also why so many of us are now addicted to carbohydrates. So don't blame yourself for your weight issues. It really isn't your fault.

When it comes to losing weight, it can all seem overwhelming. But don't get discouraged and give up, particularly when you listen to all the contradictory and conflicting advice and information you have been given throughout the years. I understand why it can make you want to scream "Enough!" However, I also want to assure you that science has caught up with much of what goes on in our bodies. We now have solid information and research that shows us that inflammation is the primary culprit in making us fat. And, most important, we now know what to do about it. So hang in there. We're going to fix all your problems with fat, but first let's talk a little bit about health and nutrition.

CHAPTER 2

ARE YOU OVERFED *AND* UNDERNOURISHED?

"The mistake is to think that if you eat an abundance of calories, your diet automatically delivers all the nutrients your body needs. But the opposite is true. The more processed food you eat, the more vitamins you need."

—MARK HYMAN, MD

▶ When talking about food, most people tend to focus primarily on macronutrients, the catchall umbrella term used to describe proteins, fats, and carbohydrates. In order to lose your FATflammation and enjoy optimal health, however, you'll also need to get enough micronutrients and phytonutrients—the vitamins, minerals, and antioxidants that keep us healthy and leave us feeling energized. Remember, the FATflammation-Free Diet Program isn't just about being skinny! Sure, you want to look great, but you also want to feel great.

Believe it or not, many people with FATflammation are also malnourished. It doesn't matter how much you weigh or how much you eat. The important question you always have to stop and ask yourself is whether you are getting all the vitamins and minerals you need to fight your fat, including trace minerals. Think about some of the diets you and/or your friends have started. Men and women trying to lose fat sometimes go to extreme lengths. They go on high-protein diets that allow no carbohydrates, cabbage soup diets that provide little or no protein, and three-day fasts that call for nothing but a drink made from lemons, water, maple syrup, and cayenne pepper.

Some dieters try to give up sugar and instead become addicted to sugar substitutes. They drink diet sodas instead of having lunch; sugar-free ice cream replaces dinner. And some men and women regularly go through times during which they reduce their caloric intake to such a degree that they feel as though they are living on air. It's also interesting to note that some animal studies suggest that a poor-quality diet, even though it's low in calories, can help create fat.

When we hear the word *malnourished,* we tend to think of poor sad children with extended bellies living in still developing countries. It seems almost unbelievable to hear that nutritional deficiencies exist in some of our most economically well-advantaged American cities, towns, and suburbs. But nutritional deficiencies are real and contribute to our problems with inflamed fat cells. A surprising number of my clients have been malnourished despite being overweight. They frequently have histories of eating too many low-nutrient refined carbohydrates, too little protein, and too few nutrient-dense foods like fruits and vegetables.

I often remember one of my clients, Greta, who described herself as the "standard, overweight middle-aged woman," though one with an autoimmune disorder. She came to me wanting to lose forty pounds. But weight wasn't her only problem; Greta was also feeling generally crummy and tired all the time. Because of her autoimmune disease Greta took her fatigue for granted. This was how she expected to feel. In the first month working together, she lost ten pounds, which was great from her point of view. Even better was the fact that she had lost her draggy sense of constant fatigue. She was so happy that she was no longer tired all the time that she wrote me a letter saying, " . . . when I noticed this, the weight loss was no longer my driving force to eat well. My health, my well-being, my body was the focus point. Losing weight was just a bonus I didn't have to pay attention to. I can't believe I'm saying this but it's true. I really did change at this point from obsessing about my weight to thinking about my state of health."

Greta did lose the forty pounds, and as her FATflammation receded, she noticed some other benefits she hadn't expected. For example, the skin on her face and arms smoothed out, and a spot of psoriasis diminished. Perhaps the most obvious change, however, showed itself on the nails on her hand. When she started on the FATflammation-Free Diet Program, one of her fingernails was heavily ridged with what are known as "beau's lines," a clear indication of malnutrition. After several months, Greta noticed that her nail was healthy and growing normally. There were no beau's lines. Like others, Greta had discovered that it is possible to be simultaneously overweight and undernourished. And that it is possible to lose weight and be well nourished.

NUTRIENT-RICH FOOD
(YES, HERE COME THE VEGGIES AND FRUITS)

I recently read a study done by University College, London. "Eating seven or more portions of fruit and vegetables a day," the study summarized in a single sentence, "reduces your risk of death at any point in time by 42 percent compared to eating less than one portion." The study, which also found that vegetables were more protective than fruit, examined the eating habits of more than 65,000 people representative of the British population during a twelve-year period, between 2001 and 2013.

Eating more fruits and veggies has an additional side benefit: many people who start eating a more nutrient-dense diet immediately notice that many of their food cravings disappear. Why would adding more green, yellow, and orange vegetables to your diet make your desire for sugar disappear? When you fail to get all the healthy nutrients you need, you will experience intense cravings, a tendency to overeat, food addictions, hunger, and poor health. It's estimated that at least 70 percent of the American diet is made up of processed foods. This means that your body is crying out for foods that will help restore balance. Vegetables and low-sugar fruits will help restore that balance. (Most vegetables are considered complex carbohydrates, while fruits are sometimes thought of as simple carbohydrates. But both fruit and vegetables contain fiber.)

If you want to win your battle against fat, you need to eat as nutrient dense a diet as possible. And the most nutrient-dense food available comes from plants. Which is why the FATflammation-Free Diet Program puts a strong emphasis on vegetables and fruits, particularly nonstarchy veggies and fruits with significantly lower sugar content.

That includes foods that are rich in . . .

Beta-carotene and other carotenoids (leafy greens, asparagus, broccoli, vegetable greens, turnips, collards, and beets, squash, spinach, as well as sweet potatoes)

Lutein (kale, spinach, and other greens)

Lycopene (tomato, watermelon, red grapefruit)

Flavonoids (onions, parsley, peppers, artichokes, berries, as well as spices such as thyme, dill, and turmeric)

Specific examples of fruits that help fight FATflammation include blueberries and blackberries, both of which are high in flavonoids as well as the antioxidant resveratrol that helps protect against heart disease and cancer, among other illnesses.

The FATflammation-Free Diet Program emphasizes those vegetables and fruits that are low in sugar and starch. For the most part, you can have as many nonstarchy vegetables as you want. You will note, however, that there are some starchy vegetables, such as white potatoes, parsnips, rutabagas, beets, and turnips, that you will asked to avoid, particularly when you first get started on the diet.

It's very easy to go overboard with fruit. The FATflammation-Free Diet Program allows two low- to moderate-sugar fruits a day, such as berries and green apples. High-sugar fruits, such as bananas, figs, grapes, watermelon, pineapple, and mangos, are not recommended. Similarly, dried fruits are incredibly high in sugar so you will really need to stay away from dried fruit such as raisins, figs, dates, and apricots.

VITAMINS, MINERALS, AND ANTIOXIDANTS

I always suggest my clients take a multivitamin each day as a foundation. There are other specific supplements that will help reverse FATflammation and help protect against inflamed fat cells; I regularly discuss these with my clients and I've included a list of recommended supplements on page 212. I am aware that there is controversy about some supplements. And most of us have heard that we should be getting our vitamins and minerals from the food we eat. I agree with this philosophy—in theory. In an ideal world, that might be true; in fact, it was probably true for our great-grandparents. But here in the twenty-first century, it's almost impossible to get all the micronutrients we need from our food. There are many reasons for this, not the least of which is that much of our food is being grown in soil that is depleted of minerals and other essential nutrients. If you want the most nutritious produce, you need healthier soil. Farmers who understand this alternate their fields, giving them time to rest. They also realize that pesticides and strong fertilizers are bad for the health of their soil. Small local farmers, many of whom are organic, usually grow produce that is higher in vitamins and minerals.

In a study published in 2004, a team of researchers from the University of Texas studied U.S. Department of Agriculture nutrition data from 1950 and 1999 for forty-three different vegetables and fruits. They found "reliable declines" in the amount of protein, calcium, phosphorus, iron riboflavin (vitamin B_2, and vitamin C. Other studies have reported the same findings. In all probability, the string bean or carrot you are eating today is simply not as rich in nutrients as it might have been in the past. Factory farming has focused on producing vegetables that are fast growing and pest resistant. This is another argument for buying as much as possible from your small local farmers.

Does all this mean that you need to take vitamin supplements? For years, some people have argued against the use of a daily multivitamin, saying that there is no study that absolutely proves that doing so is beneficial. Well, in fact there are many studies that substantiate the benefits of vitamin supplementation. A long-term study of 80,000 nurses, for example, shows that taking a multivitamin daily for fifteen years may reduce the risk of colon cancer by 75 percent!

Another study showed that 500 mg daily intake of vitamin C—taken with antioxidants beta-carotene, vitamin E, and zinc—slowed the progression of advanced age-related macular degeneration by about 25 percent and visual acuity loss by 19 percent in individuals at risk for the disease.

New research indicates also that vitamin B supplements may help reduce your risk of stroke, and a team of scientists from Harvard and Oxford, as well as other universities, found strong evidence that vitamin D protects our health. They found that men and women with lower levels of vitamin D had a 35 percent increased risk of death from heart disease and a 14 percent greater likelihood of death from cancer. Researchers also found that people who took vitamin D_3 had an 11 percent reduction in mortality from all causes. Other studies have suggested that vitamin D helps protect against diabetes and stroke.

Inflammation also shortens telomeres, the caps at the end of each strand of DNA that protect chromosomes from deterioration or prevent different strands from fusing together. They are often compared to the plastic tips on the end of shoelaces that protect your laces from fraying. As you get older, these protective telomeres get shorter. Theoretically, the longer your telomeres, the more years you can be expected to live. Longer telomeres result in healthier people and greater longevity. Telomeres that are 5 percent longer translate to a biological age ten years younger, and supplements can help lengthen your telomeres. One study of 600 women, for instance, showed the women who took multivitamin supplements had telomeres that were 5 percent longer than women who took no supplements.

Vitamins, Minerals, and Antioxidants That Fight Fatflammation

Some vitamins, minerals, and antioxidants are particularly useful in our fight against inflammation. Here's a list of some of the phytonutrients that should always be part of your life.

Vitamin A and Pro-Vitamin A

Beta-carotene is a pro-vitamin that converts to vitamin A in the body. Vitamin A is also an antioxidant that helps protect the body against free radicals. We can boost the vitamin A in our bodies by eating a wide range of vegetables including broccoli, carrots, dandelion, spinach, cantaloupe, kale, sweet potato, and collard greens.

Vitamin B

People who have low levels of vitamin B_6 tend to have high levels of C-reactive protein, which is a measure of inflammation within the body. Vegetables that are high in B vitamins, including B_6, include mushrooms, kale, broccoli, cauliflower, and bell peppers. Animal sources include turkey, chicken, cod, and tuna.

Folate (folic acid) is another B vitamin associated with inflammation. A short study in Italy suggests that even a low-dose, short-term daily folic acid supplement could reduce inflammation in people who are overweight. Good sources of folate include black-eyed peas, lima beans, chickpeas, dark leafy greens, and asparagus.

Vitamin C

A large number of studies show the anti-inflammatory benefits of foods that are high in the antioxidant vitamin C. Good lower sugar sources include tomatoes and tomato juice. You can also find vitamin C in many other fruits with a low to moderate sugar content including grapefruit and lemons. In the FATflammation-Free Diet, you start your day drinking water and lemon juice, which will give your vitamin C a morning boost.

Vitamin D

Vitamin D helps reduce inflammation and insufficient vitamin D is associated with a range of inflammatory conditions. In combination with calcium, vitamin D also promotes weight loss. There are estimates that say that two-thirds of the population in the United States is vitamin D deficient. We get vitamin D naturally when we are out in the sun. In addition, we get it in foods such as fish, egg yolks, and organ meats. It's also found in foods that have been supplemented with vitamin D, such as milk.

Vitamin E

This is another antioxidant vitamin that can help reduce inflammation. We find vitamin E naturally in nuts and seeds, including almonds and sunflower seeds, as well as in vegetables such as spinach and fruits like avocado.

Vitamin K

Vitamin K can help reduce inflammatory markers; research shows that it may help protect against heart disease, as well as osteoporosis. Very few of us are getting enough vitamin K in our diets. There are two types of vitamin K: vitamin K_1, which we find in leafy vegetables like kale, cabbage, cauliflower, and spinach; and vitamin K_2, which is found in liver and eggs.

Coenzyme Q10

This is an antioxidant that appears to have anti-inflammatory properties. We can find it naturally in sardines, mackerel, salmon, beef liver, olive oil, walnuts, peanuts, parsley, broccoli, avocado, and spinach.

Glutathione

Another antioxidant and free-radical fighter with anti-inflammatory properties (free radicals are unstable atoms or groups of atoms that can cause cell damage), glutathione can be found naturally in asparagus, avocados, spinach, garlic, tomatoes, grapefruit, apples, and milk thistle.

Magnesium

This is a mineral that can help reduce inflammation. Low magnesium is associated with high stress. Stress, as most of us know, can trigger cravings for foods such as chocolate or other refined carbohydrates. Stress also alters dopamine levels in the brain, and dopamine is a magnesium-dependent neurotransmitter. It's estimated that 70 percent of all Americans are deficient in magnesium. This is an amazing statistic because magnesium is found in a large variety of foods, including dark leafy vegetables such as spinach, avocado, almonds, and many legumes. A magnesium deficiency is particularly common among men and women who are overfat. That many of us are not getting enough of this mineral speaks to the poor quality of nourishment that exists in many of our lives.

When you realize that as many as 90 percent of adults in the United States don't get enough vitamin D or E; as many as 40 percent aren't ingesting enough vitamin C; and 50 percent are failing to get enough vitamin A, calcium, or magnesium, you realize that you could be one of these people suffering from a nutritional deficiency or, even worse, you may be malnourished.

My mother was overfed and undernourished. So was my client Greta. While my mother was never able to introduce enough micronutrients into her system, Greta was—and the results are undeniable. The key to battling fat is to eat as nutrient dense a diet as possible. But don't think that the FATflammation-Free Diet is limited only to fruits and vegetables. It's much more fun than that. It features plenty of healthy sources of meat, poultry, and fish, all of which are essential sources of fat, a surprising—and one of your most potent—ally in your battle against fat.

CHAPTER 3

FAT: THREE LITTLE LETTERS THAT CARRY A LOT OF WEIGHT

"It's simple. If it jiggles, it's fat."
—ARNOLD SCHWARZENEGGER

▶ Like Arnold Schwarzenegger, many of us are accustomed to having a simplistic view of body fat. We think of it as just a bunch of jiggly stuff around our waists, bellies, thighs, and butts. In recent years, however, science has learned a great deal about that flabby mass, and we know that it's not that simple. We now know that fat is not the inert substance we once imagined it to be. Fat, also known as adipose tissue, is now recognized as the largest endocrine organ in our bodies. This means that your fat itself is central to all issues that have to do with how you gain and lose weight. Getting a better handle on how fat works (and I don't just mean the stuff on your hips) can help you get thin.

Our fat has several primary and important functions.

1. It stores energy (in the form of calories) from the food we eat.

2. It produces and releases the hormones that control metabolism.

3. It insulates and cushions the body.

Most of the fat in our bodies is whitish in color, which is why it is known as white fat. But we each also have some brownish-colored fat. For a long time, scientists believed that brown fat was predominantly found in infants. Recently, however, they have discovered that adults also have small, almost minuscule, amounts of brown fat. For every ten pounds of white fat, for example, you're only going to have about an ounce of brown fat. Leaner people have more brown fat; so do children. Young women are going to have more brown fat than overweight older men. If you are fortunate enough to have measurable amounts of brown fat, it is typically located on the front of the neck and upper chest. Interestingly, researchers have also discovered that our brown fat is more active during the winter months when it is cold.

Experts say that brown fat is more like muscle than fat and that, when activated, it appears to be able to burn white fat. As little as three ounces may burn several hundred calories a day. There is also new evidence showing that one of the end products of exercise is an activation of brown fat. Researchers are currently trying to develop a weight-loss drug that would work by increasing and activating brown fat. The goal would be to take some of our calorie-storing white fat and turn it into calorie-burning brown fat. That would make everything a lot easier, wouldn't it? In the meantime, fighting FATflammation is the way to go.

YOUR EXPANDING AND SHRINKING FAT CELLS

We are all born with billions of fat cells, and we add billions more as we go through childhood. The average human has approximately forty billion fat cells; somebody who is obese may have as many as a hundred billion. You cannot reduce the number of fat cells in your body. You may lose thirty pounds and get "thinner," but the number of fat cells remains the same. There is some research looking at people who had weight-loss surgery or liposuction. Two years after the surgery, these men and women were typically much thinner. However, they still had the same number of fat cells.

What does change as you lose or gain weight is the size of the individual fat cells. Put on ten pounds, and your fat cells swell; put on fifty pounds, and they plump up even more, multiplying in size as many as ten times. Lose weight, and those fat cells shrink accordingly. Many people want to know whether their fat cells ever die off. Well, yes they do. Since our bodies are always making new cells, 10 percent of your fat cells die off each year; they are replaced by an equal number of new fat cells.

Scientists used to believe that individuals only accumulated additional fat cells during infancy or puberty, but new research indicates that adults can also add new fat cells. When you gain a great deal of weight as an adult, particularly if you do it in a short period of time, and your fat cells have already expanded to their fullest capacity, your body may create new fat cells.

ALL THE PLACES WHERE WE FIND FAT

You probably think that you know the precise areas in your body where fat tends to gravitate, but it may actually be in a few places you haven't considered.

Subcutaneous fat

This is the fat that is found right under your skin on your butt, hips, thighs, and belly. Pinch your thighs or your stomach. Subcutaneous fat is the fat you are holding between your fingers. Cellulite, for example, is subcutaneous fat. Subcutaneous fat may not be pretty, but it's less dangerous than visceral fat, the fat we can't see.

Visceral fat

This is the fat buried deep in our bodies, for the most part out of reach—within the abdomen, for example, filling the spaces between vital organs like the liver and kidneys. Visceral fat is linked to a multitude of major health problems including our issues with cholesterol, insulin resistance, and diabetes. Interestingly, there are some people who appear thin, but who nonetheless have a substantial amount of visceral fat hiding out around their organs and creating health concerns.

Belly Fat

The fat we all love to hate is a combination of subcutaneous and visceral fat. If you are aware of subcutaneous fat on your abdomen, it probably means that you have a fair amount of dangerous inflammatory visceral fat hiding under what you can see.

Fat Doesn't Have To Be Part of Your Genetic Heritage

I always hear people say things like, "Fat runs in my family," so I guess that's why I keep gaining weight." I grew up with a mother who had major weight issues so this is something that always concerned me. I'm thrilled to tell you that there are many new scientific discoveries, and here's what all of us who thought "fat" was part of our genetic heritage need to know.

Until very recently, we were taught that our genes determine our destiny and that our genes could not be altered or changed. The Human Genome Project showed us that this is not true. We now know that we are far more complicated than our genes. What this means is that while you may have the gene for a specific ability like artistic talent, or an illnesses like diabetes, or even a propensity to gain weight, other factors are capable of suppressing the expression of that gene. What kind of factors? Our environment, diet, and even lifestyle all make a difference in what happens with our genetic heritage. The newly emerging science of epigenetics is showing that what happens with our genes is dependent on what happens in our lives.

Essentially our genes have an "epigenome," and this epigenome sits on top of the genes. Think of your genome as being like computer hardware. If you program your computer, you don't change the hardware.

But you do change the software that tells the computer what to do.

Our genes have instructions on them via the epigenome through our lifestyle choices that essentially tell our bodies how to perform, and these genes interact with our environment. Epigenetics is showing how your environment and your choices can have a positive, or negative, influence on your genetic code. The choices we make and the experiences we have all leave a signature or mark on our genes. These signatures or marks on the gene authorize some parts of the gene to go forward and others to hold back.

To illustrate this further, think of a grand piano. The keys are like genes. They are silent until fingers on the keyboard pick out a tune (our choices). The result? A beautiful sound (positive gene expression) or sounds you don't appreciate (negative gene expression).

It turns out that we have much more control over how our genes express than we ever thought. How we influence our genes through diet, lifestyle choices, and even what we think is our key to health and happiness. In fact, science now shows that we have 80 percent control.

The Agouti Mouse Study illustrates how environmental changes can impact our genes. The Agouti mouse, which has a yellow coat color, is obese and prone to diabetes and cancer. Researchers took pregnant Agouti mice and fed them the nutrients folate, vitamin B_{12}, betaine, choline, and methionine. The baby mice then born from these obese yellow-coated unhealthy mothers were healthy, slim, and had brown coats; they were also without the Agouti gene responsible for obesity, diabetes, cancer, and a yellow coat. These results show that our health is not only determined by what we eat, but also what our parents ate.

It's interesting to know that if you make different healthier choices before you have children, your children and grandchildren will also inherit the benefits of these healthier choices in their genes. The bottom line: You can be the master of your genes!

WOMEN AND MEN STORE FAT DIFFERENTLY

Men tend to consume more calories, but women store more fat. Hormones like estrogen and testosterone make a difference in how your fat is stored. The average overweight man, for example, is likely to store fat in his abdomen, taking the form we think of as apple shaped. This abdominal fat is usually the more dangerous visceral fat.

Until she reaches menopause, the average woman is more pear shaped and tends to store mostly subcutaneous fat in her thighs, hips, and butt. Yes, there is that cellulite again. After that, as less estrogen is produced, her shape often changes and fat moves over and invades her waist and abdomen. For years we were told that pear-shaped bodies are less prone to heart disease and diabetes than those that are apple shaped. New research, however, indicates that the belief in the protective benefits of a pear shape may be more myth than reality. It turns out that weight in the hips, thighs, and butt might carry as many health hazards as it does when it is spread out around your middle.

HORMONES AND FAT

Estrogen is a fat-storing hormone, while progesterone and testosterone help our bodies release, or burn, fat. Estrogen and progesterone are thought of as a female hormones and testosterone is associated with men. However, let's start out by saying that women also make small amounts of testosterone, while men produce small amounts of estrogen as well as progesterone. Women produce estrogen primarily in their ovaries. However, some estrogen is also produced by the liver, adrenal glands, and breasts. Here's the interesting part; both men and women produce estrogen in their fat cells, a complex process that promotes excess fat.

Postmenopausal women make less estrogen and progesterone and store more fat, particularly abdominal fat, than younger women. Progesterone helps women burn off their fat. So to make matters worse for women, when their bodies start producing less progesterone, they burn off less fat. In short, all those women who say, "I gained weight after menopause even though I ate the same amount of food," are sharing an accurate report of their experience. After menopause, you do need to get more into exercise mode to budge those fat cells. I also want to assure you that I've known many, many women who have been able to do this. And I know you can be one of them. So don't get discouraged!

Men also have fat cells that create estrogen, which is a fat-storing hormone for both sexes. When men put on too much weight, causing their fat cells to expand, their estrogen levels also rise. This extra estrogen triggers the male body to make less testosterone. This can be the beginning of a vicious cycle, because the less testosterone a man produces, the more likely it is that the fat cells in his belly will expand.

Other hormones act as messengers, carrying instructions and information from one part of the body to another. The following "messenger" hormones are directly connected to your issues with fat.

Insulin

Insulin, a fat-storing hormone produced in the pancreas, makes sure that fat is stored in the fat cells. Insulin's job is to keep the amount of glucose in your blood from becoming too high. Each time you have something to eat, glucose levels in your blood rise and insulin is then released into your bloodstream. Sugar, carbohydrates, and starch create higher levels of glucose, and so your body releases higher levels of insulin. Both insulin and glucose then make their way to cells throughout the body. Insulin helps the cells absorb glucose and release it for energy. In this way, insulin keeps your blood glucose levels in check. Insulin also helps send messages that tell your liver and muscles to store glucose. When your body is functioning normally, this is a smooth process.

But some people are insulin resistant. This means that their bodies are producing insulin, but it is not doing what it should be doing. Instead of being utilized by the cells, the glucose is building up in the blood. This situation can lead to prediabetes or even type 2 diabetes. A person with type 1 diabetes has a pancreas that isn't capable of producing insulin. Type 2 diabetes means that even though your pancreas is able to make insulin, your body isn't able to use it effectively.

Glucagon

Glucagon, a fat-releasing hormone, is also produced by the pancreas, but its function is the exact opposite of the one performed by insulin. The pancreas releases glucagon when glucose levels in the blood get too low. This can happen, for example, when you skip a meal. Ideally, insulin and glucagon work together to keep your blood glucose levels balanced and stable.

Leptin

The fat cells themselves produce leptin, another fat-releasing hormone, and secrete it into the bloodstream. The name "leptin" is derived from the Greek word *lepton,* which means "thin." Leptin has a very simple message to deliver. It tells us: "You're full. Stop eating. Enough food! Enough food!" That's right, leptin reduces appetite. Its job is to tell us when to stop eating.

People with weight issues tend to have higher levels of leptin than their thinner friends, but it is less able to do its job. That's because as your fat cells get larger and larger, you can become less sensitive to what leptin is trying to tell you. In fact, you may actually become leptin resistant.

Ghrelin

Ghrelin (pronounced "grrrEllen") is a fat-releasing hormone known as the hunger hormone; it sends a message that is exactly the opposite of the one delivered by leptin. Ghrelin's message is "I'm hungry. Feed me. Feed me now!" Ghrelin's job is to make you feel hungry. A "growling" stomach is ghrelin in action. The amount of ghrelin circulating in your body goes up when you haven't eaten in a while and down after you have finished a meal. Ghrelin levels also appear to go through an uptick when you haven't slept or are under stress.

Cortisol

Cortisol, produced by your adrenal glands, is known as the "stress hormone." Cortisol, which is associated with fat storage, is usually highest in the morning and lowest around midnight. When you are under physical or psychological stress, there is a disruption of normal cortisol patterns and your body tends to make more of it. Many of us know what it is to have the munchies under these conditions.

Cortisol can increase the levels of glucose in your blood, and when it is chronically elevated, it encourages the body to store fat. It can also raise blood pressure. Cortisol levels also become elevated when you are not getting enough sleep or are having too much caffeine. Studies show that raised cortisol levels cause more visceral fat to be deposited in the abdominal area. Some experts also believe that stress and elevated cortisol are implicated in cellulite. That's because cellulite is partly a result of excess estrogen, some of which is produced by the fat tissue itself, and cortisol, like insulin, tells the body to store fat.

Thyroid Hormone

Thyroid hormone, produced by the thyroid gland, plays an important role in your health, well-being, and issues with weight gain. It helps regulate how carbohydrates, fats, proteins, and vitamins are metabolized. People who complain that they feel cold all the time probably already know that it helps regulate body temperature.

Women normally produce more thyroid hormone than men. That's because estrogen seems to render thyroid hormone less efficient. In fact, women who take thyroid hormone replacement are often told to increase the dosage when they start taking medications that include estrogen. Women are also more likely to have thyroid issues than men. If you're a woman over thirty-five, some experts estimate that you have a 30 percent possibility of developing a thyroid disorder.

Low levels of thyroid are associated with fat storage, and many more of us are currently being diagnosed with thyroid issues. The thyroid is very sensitive to chemicals and environmental toxins, all of which have increased around us. The thyroid also responds when there are nutritional imbalances or deficiencies in our diets. Too much or too little iodine, mineral deficiency from depleted soil, and an excess of dietary soy are all also cited as possible reasons for an inefficient thyroid.

CCK (Cholecystokinin)

CCK sends a message that says, "I'm full now." CCK, which helps burn and release fat, is able to do this even as you are in the middle of a meal. Fat and protein in your diet strongly stimulate the release of CCK, which is one of the reasons why meals that are higher in protein and fats and lower in carbohydrates keep us feeling full for longer periods of time. Increased levels of CCK can be found in your blood fifteen minutes after you start eating, and levels continue to be raised for several hours after you have finished. CCK also improves digestion by stimulating the production of liver bile.

Some evidence suggests that men and women who suffer from obesity may have lower levels of CCK.

Adiponectin

Although adiponectin is secreted by fat cells, levels of adiponectin are inversely associated with body fat; higher levels of adiponectin tend to correspond with lower levels of fat and vice versa. Some experts are now referring to adiponectin as the antiobesity hormone. Low levels of adiponectin also put you at higher risk of developing medical issues such as diabetes. Studies have indicated that we can raise our adiponectin levels naturally with exercise and a diet that includes fiber, monounsaturated fats, and omega-3 fatty acids. There's another good reason why we want to increase adiponectin levels: not only does the hormone help burn fat, it also helps reduce appetite. Dietary sources of adiponectin include foods that contain monounsaturated fats such as avocados, macadamia nuts, and olive oil. Exercise also helps you naturally raise adiponectin levels. There are several adiponectin supplements on the market, but I haven't seen any reliable research showing that they are effective.

Irisin

Named after Iris, the Greek messenger goddess, irisin, another fat-burning hormone, is a fascinating hormone produced in our muscles as a response to exercise. That's right, exercise itself is responsible for the creation of irisin. This hormone is different from other substances that come from muscle tissue because it seems to be able to enter the bloodstream and make its way to our fat cells. There, irisin appears capable of doing something truly remarkable: it is able to turn regular white fat cells into brown fat cells. Using muscle cells from human volunteers, scientists found that they had much higher levels of irisin in their cells after they completed a weeks-long jogging program than they did before. Remember, brown fat cells are capable of burning calories and helping you lose weight. This is a relatively new discovery and it helps us understand why exercise improves health and helps us lose weight.

WHAT EXACTLY DO FAT CELLS DO EVERY DAY?

Almost as soon as you start munching on a meal or a snack, your body goes to work converting the food you eat to glucose, a simple sugar that travels through your bloodstream. Glucose (blood sugar) is the primary food for all the cells in your body. How fast your glucose levels rise depends on the food you are eating. If your meal was high in carbohydrates, your glucose levels can start rising within fifteen minutes. Eating protein, fats, or fiber slows down the rate and level of the rise in glucose.

As the rise in glucose is taking place, your pancreas is busily producing insulin. Insulin, functioning much like the munching dots in Pac-Man, immediately starts gobbling up the glucose and delivering it to your cells. Muscle cells, brain cells, heart cells, and fat cells all need glucose to survive. But if you just finished a large carbohydrate-filled meal, your body may not be able to use all that glucose at that moment. This means that it will have to be stored for future use. Here's what happens: as soon as your body is finished with the digestive process, it sends glucose over to the liver, which converts it to fat and sends it to your waiting fat cells. That's where it will be stored in the form of free fatty acids.

When your body requires more energy, it turns to those fat cells for sustenance. The free fatty acids are released from the fat cells and sent off to the muscles where the energy is needed. If you're eating a diet that doesn't contribute to FATflammation and you're exercising regularly, your muscles are able to burn up the glucose that's being stored in your fat cells. This means that your fat cells don't have time to plump up that much and they stay relatively stable. When your fat cells let go of the free fatty acids, they shrink back.

This natural process of storing fat and burning fat is how your body was designed to work. In a perfect world, in which we all exercised regularly and ate ideal diets, this would all work perfectly. Unfortunately, most of us don't come close to eating an okay diet, much less a perfect one. As a result, few of us are able to fully benefit from the body's natural ability to burn fat. So that fat just sits around in our fat cells, producing inflammatory molecules.

Infants are born with healthy active fat cells. In all likelihood, up until the time you were in your teens and early twenties, your fat cells were efficiently able to perform their role in how calories are used, burned, and stored for future use. But perhaps you made lifestyle changes that included your diet and exercise routines. Then, everything about your body may have changed, including the way your fat cells do their jobs. With the challenges and frustrations that people encounter in their lives, many turn to food as a way to cope. Whether the emotion is anger, frustration, boredom, or loneliness, or even happiness, emotional eating rears its ugly head and the result is weight gain.

Let's take a look at some fat cells in the body of one woman. Let's call her Amanda. When Amanda was eighteen and getting ready for her high school graduation, she was accustomed to eating a balanced diet with enough protein and not too many carbohydrates. She also danced and was a high school cheerleader. She got lots of exercise so her fat cells were accustomed to swelling slightly after a meal and then quickly shrinking again. With all her activity, the fatty acids were burned up very quickly.

After high school, Amanda went off to college. That's where she started drinking apple juice and eating donuts for breakfast. For dinner almost every night, she had a pizza, a few oatmeal raisin cookies, and a soda. When she was studying late and felt hungry, she bought bags of chips out of a vending machine and ate them, while drinking a few more cans of soda. It didn't take long for Amanda's fat cells to respond to her dietary lifestyle by expanding. But Amanda was taking dance classes as well as playing tennis so many of the extra fatty acids that she started to accumulate were still heading to her muscles where they were being burned. She was putting on a little bit of weight, but the situation was still under control.

Today, Amanda is thirty-nine. She's a single mom with two children and a desk job. She feels as though she barely has enough time to brush her hair in the morning, let alone exercise. She put on weight with both pregnancies. Although she lost some of that baby weight, quite a few pounds remained. Amanda is now about thirty-five pounds heavier than she was when she headed off to college. Like many people with weight issues, Amanda has heard all the messages telling her that if she wants to lose weight, she needs to be very careful about the fat in her diet. Therefore, just about everything she eats is either no fat or low fat—that includes milk, yogurt, and cheese.

Let's watch what happens as Amanda eats her typical morning snack at her desk at work. She has a large low-fat blueberry muffin, which she cuts in half and slathers with a low-fat butter substitute. Along with her muffin, Amanda has a container of coffee into which she empties four packets of sugar. When she gets her coffee, she usually also buys a large diet soda, which she opens and starts drinking almost as soon as she finishes her coffee. Amanda acknowledges that she is addicted to caffeinated sodas. She also incorrectly believes that her artificially sweetened sodas, which always have zero calories, will not contribute to her issues with fat.

You don't need to have been trained in nutrition to notice that Amanda's snack has no protein. Nor does it contain any fiber or complex carbohydrates. It's all about sugar, starch, refined carbohydrates, sugar substitutes, and unhealthy oils.

By the time Amanda is halfway through with her muffin and coffee, her body is sending out loud and clear signals that say, "Sugar spike! Sugar spike! We need some insulin here. STAT!" Insulin quickly arrives on the scene ready to do its job. The glucose heads for the liver where it is converted to fat before making its way to her fat cells. Amanda's fat cells are no dummies. They know when they are stuffed. They respond by sending out leptin, a hormone that should be able to tell Amanda's body that she has had enough to eat. But is Amanda's body able to hear what it is being told? You would think yes, but the paradox about leptin is that when people are overweight, even though they keep producing and circulating leptin, they become leptin resistant and less able to hear the messages that are being sent.

What next? Amanda's meal was very high in sugar. The more sugar and refined carbohydrates we eat, the faster and higher the blood sugar spike. So once insulin did its job and made sure that the glucose was stored in her fat cells, Amanda experiences a steep drop in blood sugar. It's like she's on a roller coaster. One minute, her blood sugar was spiking. Now, it's crashing. Oh no! Leptin is trying to get her attention, saying, "You don't need any more food," but Amanda is totally oblivious. She doesn't have a clue about what her body is trying to tell her. Look what Amanda is doing now. She is heading to the cafeteria to see if she can find something else to eat. After all those carbs, she is experiencing a food craving. She wants even more! She hears the chant like a drumbeat, "More carbs! More carbs!"

What can I eat? she wonders. She wants to be healthy, but the cafeteria offers few healthy choices. She'll try to do the best she can. "I'll have a toasted whole wheat bagel," she says to the counter person. It looks yummy. She doesn't want to have any more fat, but she sees some little containers of strawberry jam and takes a look at the ingredient list. Strawberries and high-fructose corn syrup. *It's fruit,* she thinks. *How bad can that be?* Amanda spoons the jam over her bagel and takes a bite. What Amanda doesn't consider is that her "whole wheat" bagel is filled with sugar and refined white flour. She is busily chewing away. But those refined carbohydrates are quickly making her body send out the message for more insulin. And here it comes!

As long as Amanda continues on her high-refined-carbohydrate diet, her body will continue being bathed in insulin. This means that more and more fat is being stored. At this rate, the free fatty acids are not going to be released from her fat cells any time soon. The cells are growing bigger and bigger in order to contain everything she is feeding them. In fact Amanda's diet has left her with such stuffed fat cells that they have become chronically inflamed. Amanda has full blown FATflammation!

Blood Test That Checks for Inflammation

If you are concerned about inflammation and its implications for your health and well-being, I suggest that you ask your doctor for a simple blood test that checks your levels of C-reactive protein. This test could be done independently or included in any routine blood work your doctor orders. C-reactive protein, produced in the liver and found in the blood, rises in response to inflammation in the body. The test cannot tell you exactly where in your body you have inflammation. It rises, for example, when you have an infection anywhere and becomes normal when the infection recedes. Doctors sometimes order the test for C-reactive protein to gauge whether someone has a higher than normal risk of cardiovascular disease. They also use it to keep track of other conditions that cause inflammation. Elevated CRP levels have specifically been linked to obesity, and weight loss has been shown to decrease them.

I always ask my doctor to include the C-reactive protein test when I have my annual physical and blood work. It's good to know what the numbers are and whether a dietary adjustment is needed. Ideally, your CRP levels should be lower than 1.0mg/L. Make sure you discuss your results with your doctor, particularly if you have readings above 3.0 mg/L.

DIFFERENT KINDS OF INFLAMMATION

Inflammation, which is part of the body's immune response, is being implicated these days as a cause of diseases like cancer, heart disease, arthritis, diabetes, and everything in between. It is also a primary reason why so many of us are getting fatter.

There are three types of inflammation. The first is **acute inflammation**—or what the Greeks described as "the internal fire." Acute inflammation, which by the way isn't so "cute," makes its presence known because it hurts. We've all experienced the redness, swelling, and pain associated with acute inflammation. If you've ever had a nasty sunburn, a black-and-blue sprained ankle, a cut finger, or even a cold, then you know firsthand what acute inflammation feels like. You probably also know what it feels like to have these conditions go away. The sunburn fades, the cut heals, the cold gets better, the swelling and discoloration of the ankle disappear.

Because these physical symptoms caused you discomfort or even actual pain, you might assume that these acute inflammations were negative responses created by the body. But that's not the case. These physical responses actually help protect us. This kind of inflammation is a necessary part of the body's immune system. It protects us and helps us heal. When you cut your finger, or sprain your ankle, for example, inflammatory molecules in the body or "soldiers" if you will, immediately rush to the site, surround the area that was injured, and work to help heal the injury. Once the injury is healed, and the threat of infection disappears, the inflammatory molecules, or soldiers, retreat to base camp, ready to be called upon anytime in the future when the body is under attack.

But what happens if the soldiers fail to retreat? What happens if all those inflammatory molecules stay right where they are? Easy answer: the inflammation remains and doesn't go away. This leads to a condition known as **silent**, or **chronic, inflammation**. Acute inflammation is like a big tidal wave that does its damage and then settles down; silent inflammation is like the trickle from a leaking dam that may eventually burst. Chronic, or silent, inflammation describes a situation in which the inflammation stays there 24/7, doing its dirty work, without your being aware of it. Chronic inflammation is like having a sore on the inside of your body that never heals.

What's the difference between acute and silent inflammation? Acute inflammation can be compared to a raging forest fire that quickly burns through the forest and is extinguished. Silent inflammation behaves more like the smoldering embers lying in wait under the forest fire's ruins. You don't even see them, but they are there ready to burst into flames. Most of the time, you don't even know a dangerous fire is smoldering underneath the surface, waiting to happen.

Do You Have FATflammation?

Consider the following questions:

Are you overweight?

Do you feel as though your weight is out of control?

Are you seeing fat in places in the body where you never had fat before?

Do you feel bloated, particularly in the evening?

Are you retaining water—feet, ankles, belly, or fingers?

Do you have cellulite?

Do you have diabetes or prediabetes?

Do you drink fewer than eight glasses of plain water a day?

Is your fasting blood sugar on the high side of normal? (Normal range is 70–100 mg/dl.)

Are you suffering from some form of digestive problem (gas, heartburn, reflux, constipation, diarrhea) that seems to be directly in response to what you eat?

Do you eat sugar and refined carbohydrates every day?

Do you crave sugar and refined carbohydrates?

Are you sensitive or actually allergic to certain foods (wheat, dairy, soy)?

Once you start eating, do you have a difficult time stopping?

Do you get hungry within an hour or two of finishing a meal?

Are most of your meals carbohydrate centered?

Are you chronically stressed?

Are you sleep deprived?

Do you drink four or more sodas, including diet soda, a week?

Do many of the foods you eat include High Fructose Corn Syrup? (HFCS)

Do you regularly eat food prepared with omega-6 oils—corn, peanut, soybean, safflower, canola?

Do you eat in fast-food restaurants more than once a month?

Do you regularly use margarine or butter substitutes?

Does your diet include a lot of soy products?

Are you exercising less than two hours a week?

If you answered yes to more than three of these questions, the chances are that you have FATflammation, which is the core cause of weight gain. The good news is that by changing what you eat, you can reverse the insidious process taking place in your fat cells, and you can start doing it with your very next bite.

The third type of inflammation is **FATflammation**. This is a chronic silent, and dangerous, inflammation that is taking place in the fat cells themselves. Your body has had to deal with so much unhealthy food, such as Omega-6 vegetable oils, sugar, High Fructose Corn Syrup, trans fats, refined carbohydrates in the form of white rice, as well as pasta and bread made with modern wheat (and much more) that your fat cells themselves are experiencing a form of silent inflammation.

Your fat cells are storing energy in the form of fatty acids, which is exactly what they are supposed to do, but they have taken in so much they have become toxic and sick. Your fat cells are behaving as though they are suffering from a chronic infection; they are responding by producing inflammatory molecules.

Fat cells essentially operate in their own world—their own environment. In short, the fat cells themselves instigate an inflammatory response and, like factories, spew out inflammatory cytokines—chemical messengers that put inflammation in motion throughout the body. Not only does this make us "overfat," it negatively affects our overall health. Some of these cytokines, for example, are responsible for insulin resistance.

FATflammation may cause only a small rise in inflammatory markers, but it is chronic—24/7. The insidious highlight of FATflammation is that it is perpetual and never-ending. It becomes an inflammatory cascade. Unless you break this vicious cycle, you are not going to be able to lose weight. Even worse, your inflamed fat cells could make you sick as well as tired.

The FATflammation–Cellulite Connection

A few years back, I received a call from Gillian, an incredibly fit thirty-year-old who was accustomed to spending much of her day in a gym or on a mat working out. That's because Gillian is a fitness trainer. She spends more hours bending, stretching, squatting, and sprinting in a week than many people do in a year. Gillian was very thin, but she had two areas of concern about her body. She had belly fat that wouldn't give up, no matter how much she exercised, and she had cellulite on the back of her thighs. Cellulite, as most of us know too well, is what happens when little globs of fat deposit themselves right under the skin. When I looked at the graceful and slender Gillian, I realized that she was living proof that just about all women have cellulite. It is estimated that 90 percent of all women (from the very thinnest to the most overfat) have some of that lumpy, bumpy, pitted skin known as cellulite, forming not-so-cute dimples on all those places where women naturally store fat, such as thighs, hips, and butts. Although some men have cellulite, for the most part, it's a female issue. There are two reasons for this:

1. Estrogen

   After puberty, women experience a natural surge of estrogen, sending a signal to their bodies to store fat.

2. Connective tissue

   These are the fiberlike substances under the skin that connect skin to muscle. Connective tissue in men forms in a crisscross pattern—think of a fish net. This creates a barrier that helps keep the fat from bumping up against the skin. Women's connective tissue, on the other hand, forms in parallel lines like a picket fence, giving those little fat cells we call cellulite a way to slip through and push up to the skin where they become very noticeable.

In this country, fighting cellulite is a multimillion-dollar industry. Women concerned with cellulite are trying everything available and spending a fortune while they are doing it. Here's a list of some of the current cellulite treatments: topical creams, lotions, potions, retinoic acid, laser treatments, radio frequency ablation, regular massage, liposuction, deep tissue massage, body wraps, along with a variety of externally applied herbal extracts and botanicals such as algae, plankton, butcherbroom ginger root, cinnamon, green tea, and capsaicin, ginkgo biloba, evening primrose oil, sweet clover, grapeseed oil, not to mention coffee grounds, and, even hormone treatments such as progesterone.

Does any of it work? Some people say yes; others say no. One of the reasons why it's difficult to give informed answers about the success rate of various treatments for cellulite is that there has been minimal careful scientific research. Science does not regard cellulite as a disease, and it's not. But it sure is unpleasant, and we sure don't like the way it looks. (By the way, don't confuse cellulite with cellulitis, which is a serious bacterial infection.)

All the factors that create FATflammation are also implicated in cellulite. Think dehydration, sluggish metabolism, liver overload, insulin resistance, too many omega-6 and too few omega-3 fatty acids. And we absolutely do know that cellulite is connected to our problems with fat. Women who suffer from inflamed fat cells and FATflammation tend to have more cellulite. I've had a large number of clients whose cellulite started disappearing as soon as their fat cells started shrinking. I remember one client, Debra, who was particularly concerned with her cellulite. Yes, she wanted to lose weight, but she appeared even more eager to get rid of her cellulite. "I just hate it," she said. And the cellulite on her thighs, from her knees to her butt, was quite noticeable.

Debra went on the FATflammation-Free Diet Program to reverse her fat cell inflammation. She also began taking the recommended supplements (including omega-3 fish oil) and within four weeks, she was well on her way to reaching her desired weight. What made her happiest, however, was the reduction in her cellulite. It had changed texture and become difficult to see. She also said that the skin on her thighs had become "softer" and lost that dry cellulite look. She shrunk her fat cells while removing the toxic buildup within them, and the omega-3 fats, which had been added to her diet, exerted a direct anti-inflammatory effect on the fat cell itself. This presented with weight loss and less dimpling.

I have also seen clients whose cellulite appeared to be directly related to food sensitivity and often they had not been aware of their sensitivity. If someone eats a food to which she is sensitive, the body becomes inflamed, and a cascade of hormonal events occurs, such as increased cortisol and insulin and leptin resistance. In the end, weight gain occurs. My client Gillian, for example, was sensitive to gluten. She was finally able to connect the dots between what she was eating and how she felt. Gillian, who was thin except for her belly fat and cellulite on her thighs, was able to lose her cellulite by going on the FATflammation-Free Diet Program, balancing her omega-3/omega-6 fatty acids, and addressing her food sensitivity by removing gluten from her diet.

By following the principles of the FATflammation-Free Diet Program, you will quickly and swiftly reverse FATflammation and take control of your issues with weight. Fat holds on to toxins, which is one of the primary reasons why you feel sluggish and tired, as well as fat. By following the FATflammation-Free Diet Program, you will take care of your problems with insulin sensitivity, trigger the hormones that raise your metabolism, detox your liver, and reduce the toxins in your body. Taking the recommended actions will set off a cascade of cellular events that will shrink your fat cells and leave you leaner and healthier, as well as more energized. What's not to love about that?

PART TWO

GETTING RID OF FATFLAMMATION: YOUR GAME PLAN

CHAPTER 4

BREAK UP WITH THE FATFLAMMATION FOUR

*"I always knew that if I wanted to get rid of my fat, I would
have to stop eating bread, pasta, and sugar. And I made
many halfhearted attempts to do just that. But I would
usually end up giving up only bread or only sugar, and
I would only do it for a day or two. Finally, I decided that I
couldn't fool around with my plans to lose weight any longer.
The time had come. I was planning a huge birthday party
for my boyfriend. Lots of people I hadn't seen in years were
going to be there. So I did it. I went cold turkey. No sugar, no
pasta, no bread! Once I made up my mind, it wasn't even
that difficult. Within five days—I am not exaggerating—
my clothes started to feel looser and close women friends
began to ask me what I was doing to lose weight."*

—MEGAN

▶ Breaking up is hard to do. But you recognize that the relationship you
have with food is no longer working. You hate the way you look; you hate the
way you feel. The time has definitely come to do something about it! Here's
the tough part: if you want to get your inflamed fat cells back down to size,
you have to stop eating the foods that make your fat cells behave as though
they are infected.

Take a long hard look at the following list. When it comes to losing weight, these are your most powerful enemies. I have no reservations about telling you how damaging these substances are to your health, as well as your weight. The newest studies definitely show that foods containing these ingredients inflame your fat cells and cause FATflammation.

The FATflammation Four

1. Sugar

2. Refined grains

3. High-fructose corn syrup

4. Artificial sweeteners

I understand that the idea of giving up so many of your favorite foods might seem daunting. I know that you worry that you will feel deprived; I know that you wonder what you will be able to eat; I know that you think you will feel hungry all the time; I know that you are concerned that you won't be able to do it. So, before we go any further, I just want to reassure you that I am absolutely certain that you are capable of breaking up with the foods that are making you fat as well as playing havoc with your health. *You can do it!*

FATFLAMMATION ENEMY NUMBER ONE: SUGAR

Few Americans can get through the day without some form of sugar. Recently I went to breakfast at a local restaurant and, as soon as we sat down, the waiter brought us a platter of assorted three-by-three-inch squares of assorted breads and cakes. It was a huge pile of zucchini breads, ginger breads, corn breads, and cranberry breads. The first thing that went through my head was, *This is really unhealthy!* I started thinking about all the hungry people around me in the restaurant, who hadn't eaten all night, and were now ordering breakfast. The very first morsel of food that most of them would be putting into their bodies was sugar and white flour—CAKE, essentially. Nearly everyone in the restaurant—men, women, and children—had some sort of sweet on their plates.

And lest you start to think that this was a rare instance of overindulgence, here are some scary facts: In the early 1800s, the average American ate approximately 2 pounds of sugar per year. Back then, sugar served only as an occasional treat; it wasn't a staple of the American diet. But as our country grew, so did our sugar consumption, year by year, decade by decade. By the early 1970s, Americans, on average, gobbled up approximately 123 pounds of sugar per year. Today, our average yearly sugar consumption is more than 150 pounds per person, or more than 42 teaspoons of sugar per person, per day. That's a whole lot of sugar, which triggers a whole lot of insulin, which creates a whole lot of inflammation, which leads to a whole lot of fat!

A few years back, Dr. Robert Lustig, a leading expert in childhood obesity at the University of California, San Francisco, gave a ninety-minute lecture called "Sugar: The Bitter Truth." The video was later posted on YouTube; it quickly went viral. Dr. Lustig warned us that sugar is not just an empty calorie and that its effect on our health and well-being is much more insidious. "It's not about the calories," he said. "It has nothing to do with the calories. It's a poison by itself."

There is no way around it: sugar is your first-class ticket to FATflammation. Put a couple of teaspoons of sugar in your coffee or tea, give it a stir, start drinking, and here's what happens: the amount of glucose in your blood starts going up, up, up. Your body, then, self-protectively releases insulin to lower your blood sugar. When this happens, insulin, a very powerful hormone, tells your body, "START STORING FAT!" And your body does just that. The more sugar you ingest, the higher your blood glucose rises; and the higher your blood glucose rises, the more insulin your body produces. And as your body produces more and more insulin, the more fat it stores. That's why you need to break up with sugar.

Even though we might understand mentally that we need to break up with sugar, we can never quite bring ourselves to end it once and for all? Why? Why is it so hard to break up with sugar? Well, how about because IT'S EVERYWHERE! If you go to work, how do you avoid the coffee breaks and the donuts, and the office parties, or the woman down the hall who keeps bringing in homemade fudge? What do you do when a friend invites you to her house for coffee and offers you a tray of homemade banana bread along with a bowl of fruited yogurt that is more sweetened syrup than yogurt? What do you do when friends have a birthday party for you and one of them has baked a luscious-looking orange cake with chocolate frosting? Do you hurt her feelings by refusing to have a piece? And what about all those holidays filled with sweet goodies! You remember how much you loved Halloween as a child. Today, as an adult, you probably still want to give out candy to the neighborhood kids. How can you manage to do that without popping at least one little Reese's Peanut Butter Cup into your mouth? And we also know that once you have one, you can't stop.

What kind of relationship do you have with sugar? Just how close are you? Can you take it or leave it? Or is sugar your go-to best friend whenever you feel sad, lonely, or just a little bored? Have you ever described yourself as a "sugar junkie"? How about a "chocoholic"? Or a "candy addict"? Did you ever go to the store, buy a package of cookies, and eat every single one before you got home? For that matter, can you keep cookies or candy in your home without eating them all up, sometimes before anybody else even knows they are there? How about ice cream? If there is a pint, or even a quart, of ice cream in your freezer, do you devour it, sometimes in one sitting? And let's not forget about soda. Can you get through a day without your soda "fix"?

Many of us joke about being sugar addicts. But we think it's a joke, right? Sure, we've all read reams about all the ways in which sugar is harmful to our bodies. We may even acknowledge that it is probably toxic (even as we keep eating it), but do we truly accept that it is genuinely addictive? The latest research tells us that our constant desire or craving for sugar may be more than just a "sweet tooth" issue. Research now makes it very clear: **SUGAR IS AN ADDICTIVE SUBSTANCE.**

Take The Test:
Are You Really a Sugar Addict?

What's your relationship to sugar? Here are some questions to help you form an honest answer.

Do you eat some type of food (cookies, candy, soda, cake, sweetened dry cereal, muffins, jam, jelly) that contains refined sugar every single day?

Do you find it very challenging to go more than a few hours without eating something that includes sugar?

Do you regularly have strong sugar cravings, particularly at certain times of the day?

Have you ever hidden candy, cookies, or cake around the house so nobody else will know how many sweets you are really eating?

Do you have an almost impossible time eating only one piece of candy or one bite of dessert?

When there are no other sweets in the house, have you ever found yourself eating spoonfuls of a sugar-filled substance such as jam, jelly, or chocolate syrup?

Do you feel a strong need to have something sweet after every meal?

Do you always put one or more teaspoons of sugar in your coffee or tea?

Do you drink a soda almost every day?

If there is a supply of candy, cookies, or other sweets in the house, do you find it extremely difficult not to eat them?

If you answered yes to more than four of these questions, then in all probability, you are addicted to sugar and you need to break away from it. And you need to do it TODAY!

When we think about addictive substances, we normally assume we're talking about the well-documented drugs of abuse, such as nicotine, alcohol, cocaine, heroin, or prescription pain killers. Men and women who indulge in any of these regularly are thought of as addicts because they have a compulsive need for toxic substances on which they have become dependent. There are specific behaviors that are traditionally associated with dependency: bingeing or increased use of the substance, particularly after a time of abstinence; withdrawal, characterized by anxiety or discomfort when the substance is not available; and craving, reflecting an intense need to have some of the addictive substance.

More Bad News: Sugar Causes Wrinkles

My friend Wendy lives in New England. I love Wendy for her sense of humor and positive personality. But when I called her on what she described as a blustery October afternoon, her mood was far from upbeat. A recent divorce had left her struggling with some tough challenges. She was exhausted and stressed, just kind of beaten down. She complained that her energy was so low that she didn't want to go anywhere. As a result, she was basically living an almost reclusive life. Wendy realized she needed to do more to improve her social life and start connecting with others, but it was apparent that she was uncomfortable about doing this. Why was she so reluctant to get out and be part of the world? What was holding her back? These are easy questions to answer: Wendy was upset about the weight she had gained in the last years of her marriage; she didn't feel good about herself or how she looked in clothes. She was embarrassed about letting old friends see her with the extra pounds and was worried that any potential new friends would judge her based on how she looked. Consequently, she spent most of her time at home, wearing baggy clothing and stretchy fabrics.

"Nothing fits," Wendy complained. "And it's no fun going shopping when you look like a truck."

Wendy was stuck. Because she works from home, her lifestyle was much too sedentary. She was also finding the idea of dieting overwhelming. Wendy knew about nutrition and was very careful about the meals she prepared for her children. For herself, however, she was far more likely to just reach into her refrigerator or cabinets and grab something that was overloaded with bad fats or sugar.

"Hi, Wendy, what are you doing?" I asked when she first picked up the phone.

"I'm just sitting here drinking a glass of red wine and scarfing down some Twinkies."

I groaned ever so slightly. I thought it was under my breath, but Wendy heard it.

"The Twinkies are pink—to match the wine," she said. "Does that make it better?"

"Oh, Wendy," I said. "You have to stop eating that stuff. It causes inflammation."

It was Wendy's turn to groan. "I know. I know," she said. "But right now, I'm happy here with my wine, my Twinkies, and my dog. Let me have a little fun."

I care about Wendy, and I recognized that, like most of us, she cares about how she looks, so I didn't hesitate to resort to some true scare tactics. "Sugar caramelizes body tissue—even your skin. That means it causes wrinkles and sagging. How does that work for you?!"

"Wrinkles!!! That got Wendy's attention.

I hope it does the same for you. If you have any remaining reservations about breaking up with sugar, here's something else you need to know: Not only is sugar bad for your weight and your health, it's also bad for your skin. We now know that sugar in our bloodstream attaches itself to protein molecules, including collagen and elastin, in your skin. When sugar attaches to these protein molecules, it creates destructive new molecules known as advanced glycation end products (appropriately called AGES). Anyone who has ever read a beauty magazine or looked at cosmetic ingredient lists knows that collagen and elastin help give skin that firm and youthful look. When glycation starts, so do wrinkles.

Recently scientists at Princeton University set up a laboratory experiment to see whether lab animals fed sugar would, indeed, become sugar dependent. It's not going to come as a surprise to anyone who has ever kept a stash of candy hidden away someplace in the back of a hall closet, "just in case," that the animals did, indeed, end up with full-blown sugar addictions. Research also shows that eating sugar results in a release of brain chemicals creating a rush of pleasure that is similar to what addicts get when they inject heroin.

I know what it's like to be addicted to sugar. My mother, who died when I was a teenager, was a recognizable sugar addict with serious health problems. I saw how she turned to sugar as a comfort food. When I was a young girl, I also felt as though I had to have a sugar "fix" every day. Candy was another weakness, particularly caramels, Butterfingers, and hard candy. After my mother died, I was determined to get healthier, so I turned my back on sugar with some success, despite the occasional relapse.

So now that we know that sugar addiction is real, what do you do next? Before you go any further, I'd like to ask you to repeat again: "SUGAR IS MY ENEMY."

FATFLAMMATION ENEMY NUMBER TWO: REFINED GRAINS

The very first time I met Marla, she said to me, "I don't understand why I keep gaining weight. I'm not eating that many calories."

"Make a list of everything you ate yesterday," I suggested.

"Let's see," she said, "for breakfast, I had orange juice, coffee, and a bagel. I didn't put any butter or cream cheese on the bagel. It was just a bagel. Then midmorning, I had a piece of toast with a little bit of strawberry jam—maybe half a teaspoon, and a cup of tea. For lunch: a kaiser roll, a tomato, and a piece of cheese. In the middle of the afternoon, I had a couple of small packages of oyster crackers that were in my desk—you know, the kind they give you with soup. I had nothing else until I got home. Then, for dinner, I ate a bowl of pasta with marinara sauce." Then she confessed, "Okay, I admit it. It was closer to a bowl and a half. I also ate a side salad and a couple of pieces of garlic bread. Before I went to bed, I was still hungry so I had a toasted English muffin—and a couple of tablespoons of cottage cheese. That's it."

She continued, "Come on, I didn't have that many calories and I don't eat that much sugar."

She's right. When you add up all Marla's calories from one day, it doesn't seem possible that she keeps gaining weight. What is going on? Marla is living proof that you can't use a calorie count to figure out what creates fat. In Marla's case, it is easy to see that most of her diet is made up of refined-grain products. Refined grains, such as white flour and white rice, are grains that have had the bran and germ removed during the milling process, something manufacturers do to give the grains the finer texture that most food consumers now expect. Milling also extends shelf life. Unfortunately, milling also removes much of the grain's fiber and nutritional value.

In Marla's case, it seems apparent that all those refined grains are making her fat. And here's why: REFINED GRAINS ARE METABOLIZED LIKE SUGAR. That's because they are not whole foods. They are missing fiber and other key nutrients that would normally slow down the release of sugar into the bloodstream. When you eat refined grains, your body responds as though it is getting sugar. This means that your blood glucose level takes off on a roller-coaster ride, spiking superhigh and then taking a precipitous and inflammatory drop. Remember your mantra: SUGAR IS MY ENEMY! Which means refined grains are also your enemy. Why? Because once again, your body is getting that same old message: STORE FAT! How much fat? Well, two slices of most breads, including those labeled whole wheat, can have the same kind of impact on the body as approximately seven to ten teaspoons of sugar.

Do your food preferences resemble Marla's? Do you find it more difficult to turn away from a plate of spaghetti than you do from a candy bar? Do you love all that white-on-white stuff like bread, pasta, and white rice? If that's the case, you are probably struggling with FATflammation.

It's not going to come as any surprise to learn that products made with white flour, such as bread and pasta, are the most commonly eaten foods in the United States. We love our pasta. And it's difficult for many people to understand why they are now being told to give up the bread and pasta. For many years, they were told not only that it was okay to fill up on carbohydrates, but that it was desirable.

In the famous Food Guide Pyramid, which was first issued in 1992, the largest part of the pyramid was made up of grains and cereals. Believe it or not, we were advised to consume six to eleven servings of bread, cereal, rice, and pasta a day. Let's repeat that: six to eleven servings of bread, cereal, rice, and pasta a day. When you look at that food pyramid, you will see that very little or no distinction was made between brown rice (a whole-grain product) and white rice (a refined product). Most nutritional advice at the time centered on the belief that "fat was bad." So long as we weren't eating butter, hamburgers, chops, or well-marbled steak, it was okay; when it came to carbohydrates, we were all pretty much given a free pass. I remember watching people on television saying things like, "If you don't eat any fat, how can you get fat?" Runners and athletes were advised to "carb up" before races and athletic events, and we would watch them chowing down on bagels or huge bowls of macaroni. This was considered healthy! Let me just tell you that refined grains are not healthy.

Refined grain products are plant-based foods from which the whole grain has been extracted during processing. The process of refining a grain not only removes the fiber, it also removes much of the food's nutritional value, including B-complex vitamins, healthy oils, and fat-soluble vitamins. Some of these foods have been so refined that food manufacturers are required to add nutrients back in, and the nutrients added back in are synthetic, not in their natural form. Take a look at the label on an average box of pasta or cold breakfast cereal. You will see that the ingredients include several B vitamins. These were put back as synthetic B vitamins because the natural ones contained in whole grains were stripped out during the refining process. I also want to remind you that when you go to the supermarket, you may pick up a loaf of brown-looking stuff and assume it is a healthier whole wheat. Not true. Much of the time, all you are getting is a product made of refined grains to which molasses has been added for coloring.

Are You Addicted to Refined Grains?

If you are addicted to refined grains, I'm sure you know it. But if you have any questions about it, take the following test and see if it sounds like you.

Is a plate of pasta and a hunk of garlic bread, maybe with a small side salad, your idea of a perfect meal?

Do you feel deprived if your breakfast doesn't include toast, a bagel, a muffin, or some other food made from a refined grain?

An hour or two after you've finished dinner, do you find yourself in the kitchen eating bread, pasta, rice, crackers, or some other form of refined carbohydrates?

When you have pasta for dinner, do you find the recommended serving of four ounces much too small?

Do you often fail to include a protein with your meals and/or snacks?

Once you start eating bread, do you find it difficult to stop?

Do you sometimes go through an entire day eating meals that are almost totally composed of refined carbs?

Do you regard food made with refined grains as your primary comfort food?

If you answered yes to two or more of these questions, then you need to acknowledge that you are addicted to refined grains. The time has come for you to start making better food choices. The good news about breaking up with refined grains is that there are dozens of delicious whole-grain products waiting to replace them. (We'll learn more about some of these choices in the section on complex carbohydrates.)

FATFLAMMATION ENEMY NUMBER THREE: HIGH-FRUCTOSE CORN SYRUP

"The goal of the corn industry is to call into question any claim of harm from consuming high fructose corn syrup and to confuse and deflect by calling their product natural 'corn sugar.' That's like calling tobacco in cigarettes natural herbal medicine."

—Dr Mark Hyman (*"5 Reasons High Fructose Corn Syrup Will Kill You"*)

Also known as corn sugar, high-fructose corn syrup (HFCS) is a primary—and powerful—source of FATflammation. HFCS is so bad for you, it may even be more damaging to your weight (and health) than old-fashioned cane sugar. Cane sugar and corn sugar are not the same. Both are bad, but HFCS is worse. It triggers big spikes in our insulin, sending the signal that tells our bodies to start storing fat. HFCS is also transported directly to the liver, where it is quickly metabolized, damaging the liver in a way that's similar to what happens with alcohol and other toxins.

How did HFCS become something that most of us started eating without even knowing what it was or that it was in our food? Starting back in the 1970s, the food industry powers that be decided that they would begin replacing sugar with this sweet-corn-derived additive and industrial food product. They had reasons for doing so: it was much less expensive and tasted just about as good as sugar. The name also seemed very reassuring to consumers. Many of us saw the word *fructose* and thought, *Fructose is fruit, right? That's gotta be good for you.* Well, anyone who thinks that is wrong, wrong, wrong. Since then, between 1970 and 1990, there was a 1,000 percent increase in the use of high-fructose corn sweetener in the United States. Interestingly, during this same time period, there was also a decrease in the consumption of sucrose, or table sugar. Currently, an estimated 7 percent of our daily caloric consumption comes from HFCS.

While I'm sure the food industry didn't intentionally set out to make consumers ill or fat by including HFCS in so many foods, many experts now sincerely believe that it is dangerous. Weight gain, as well as many other serious illnesses, such as diabetes, heart disease, liver disease (including fatty liver), and hypertension, are directly connected to the increased consumption of HFCS. A study conducted at UC Davis, California showed that volunteers on a diet of high levels of fructose increased the risk of heart disease, increased lipid levels, decreased insulin sensitivity, and increased levels of fat surrounding the heart and liver. Similarly, a study conducted at Princeton showed that rats given access to HFCS gained significantly more weight than animals given equal access to sucrose, even though both groups consumed the same number of total calories.

If you start reading your ingredient labels, you will discover that HFCS is included in all kinds of food and beverages products. Do not take chances with your health or your weight. I strongly recommend that you **never, ever, buy any food product that includes high-fructose corn syrup**. Also go through your kitchen, read all the labels, and toss out any HFCS products you've already purchased. I don't want to confuse you, but as you are doing this, you may notice another ingredient known as plain old-fashioned "corn syrup." Although "corn syrup" is also inflammatory, it is different from HFCS and currently used less frequently. Still, if you want to be FATflammation free, neither ingredient belongs in the food you eat.

Some responsible health-conscious food manufacturers have already started removing HFCS from their products. If you have any question about a product, you can easily check on the Internet or call the manufacturer. The food business is a multibillion-dollar industry so don't expect all companies that use HFCS to go down without a fight. They are spending a fortune trying to convince consumers that HFCS products are safe. However, research shows that HFCS is toxic to your health, particularly your liver, and a top trigger for FATflammation.

The problem with HFCS is that it is ubiquitous. It is in everything. So examine all your labels carefully. Here are some examples of food products that may include HFCS:

Breakfast cereals

Salad dressings and mayonnaise

Steak sauces and marinades

Spaghetti sauce

Ketchup

Beverages including popular sodas and many juice drinks

Cakes, cookies, candies

Soups

A wide variety of popular breads, crackers, cookies, English muffins, and stuffing mixes

Dairy products such as flavored yogurts, cottage cheese, whipped dessert toppings, and ice cream

Jams, jellies, relishes, and fruit sauces

Apple, cranberry, and other fruit sauces

Canned fruit

Baked beans, pickles, pickle relish

Chocolate, maple, and other syrups

Cough syrups, cough drops, and breath mints

Once again, read all your labels carefully. Avoid all products that include high-fructose corn syrup or corn sugar.

If you want to get rid of FATflammation, you have to say a very loud NO to HFCS.

Keeping Your Liver Healthy

Your liver's primary role is to detoxify your body. When toxins and unhealthy chemicals, such as pesticides, come your way, your liver jumps in to protect you. Think of it as a terrifically efficient washing machine. It takes in everything you consume, washes and cleans it out, then removes toxins. It does this day in and day out. Your liver takes care of you; you need to take care of it.

Your liver is also your body's number one fat-burning organ. When it comes to weight gain and loss, this is an important job. When you eat too much of the wrong thing, your liver is assaulted by your wrong choices and you end up with liver overload. If you are going to be happy, healthy, and free of FATflammation, you need a strong healthy liver.

More and more Americans are going to their doctors, having routine blood tests, including one for liver function, and discovering to their surprise that they have something described as a nonalcoholic fatty liver. For years, medical professionals associated fatty liver with people who drank too much liquor. The bodies of these heavy drinkers had been assaulted with so much alcohol that their livers could no longer deal with it. For these people, alcohol had become a toxic substance, leaving them with fat deposits within the liver itself. Discovering that heavy drinkers had liver problems was no surprise; it was to be expected.

But what explains the growing number of people who drink little or no alcohol and who are now being diagnosed with similar liver issues? It's estimated that as many as seventy million adults may be struggling with nonalcoholic fatty liver. It's also very troubling that many don't even know they have it. Fatty liver even happens to children! It is now estimated that one out of ten children in the United States (approximately seven million children) have fatty livers. How is that for a terrifying statistic? For a while, it was thought that fatty liver in children was specifically associated with obesity. But it seems to be increasing even among children without weight concerns. What could be causing this? The most obvious explanation: something in the American diet is causing this problem. Our livers are regarding something we are eating regularly as a toxic substance.

What are the food choices that put you at risk for fatty liver? It's no surprise that some of the same foods that cause FATflammation are seen as being implicated in nonalcoholic fatty liver, particularly foods containing HFCS.

When you see the term "nonalcoholic fatty liver," it's easy to assume that the culprit behind the disease is "fat." But that's not what's happening. Fat forms in the liver because of excessive amounts of sugar and refined carbohydrates. In other words, HFCS, sugar, and other refined carbohydrates can be just as toxic as alcohol.

The best examples of truly fatty livers are seen in those poor geese, force-fed corn so that their livers will fatten up and become the gourmet appetizer, foie gras. These geese are not on a diet of sirloin and butter! They are on mostly vegetarian diets and usually being fed huge amounts of corn. So does this mean that all those Americans, young and old, who are being diagnosed with nonalcoholic fatty liver disease are sitting out in midwestern cornfields gnawing away 24/7? Of course not. But there is a common element: all that corn being used to make HFCS. Children, in particular, are drinking more and more fruit beverages and sodas that include HFCS. Many medical researchers strongly believe that the introduction of HFCS into the American diet is directly linked to higher rates of obesity as well as nonalcoholic fatty liver. I find the evidence that this is the case very persuasive and recommend the following actions.

Immediately eliminate all foods that contain HFCS. This is a nonnegotiable. Read your labels.

Stop eating refined carbohydrates like sugar and anything that includes white flour.

Bring on all those vegetables high in sulfur because they help detoxify the liver. Vegetables high in sulfur include broccoli, brussels sprouts, cabbage, cauliflower, collard greens, kale, garlic, onions, and asparagus.

Consider taking two specific supplements: milk thistle, which has been shown to support liver health, and alpha-lipoic acid. I recommend that my clients take 150 milligrams of milk thistle daily and 400 milligrams of alpha-lipoic acid daily. Don't be confused and buy alpha-linoleic acid. Both alpha-lipoic acid and alpha-linoleic acid are referred to as ALA, but they are very different supplements.

Make sure you are getting all the B vitamins you need. I recommend that my clients take a daily B complex vitamin (100 mg daily).

Oils that help you fight FATflammation may also help keep your liver healthy. These include omega-3 fatty acids, olive oil, macadamia nut oil, and coconut oil.

FATFLAMMATION ENEMY NUMBER FOUR: ARTIFICIAL SWEETENERS

I meet many people who honestly believe they are doing a "good" thing by substituting artificial sweeteners for sugar. In fact, 30 percent of American adults regularly choose artificial sweeteners. If you are one of them, I want to make it very clear that you have been misled.

In the last twenty-five years, it has become fairly common for both men and women to try to cut calories and/or reduce the risk of type 2 diabetes by using artificial sweeteners. When they hit the grocery store, they choose artificially sweetened ice cream and candy. They buy artificially sweetened desserts, jams, yogurt, and syrup. They search long and hard for these items.

The most common artificial sweeteners are acesulfame potassium, aspartame, neotame, saccharin, and sucralose. They sound more familiar when we identify them with names like Equal, Splenda, NutraSweet, Sweet'N Low, Sunett, and Sweet One. These sweeteners are called "artificial" because they are chemically manufactured; they do not exist in nature. They are all many, many times sweeter than old-fashioned sugar. Aspartame, for example, is about two hundred times sweeter than sugar. Although many people use these artificial sweeteners for baking or to stir into their tea or coffee, artificial sweeteners are probably most widely used in diet soda.

While many people continue to seek out artificial sweeteners as a healthy alternative to sugar, we're just now starting to figure out their short- and long-term health consequences. Over the years, many people have started to raise questions about the possible dangers associated with artificial sugar substitutes. And the answers are less than encouraging. A number of experts, for instance, now say that the rise in obesity is connected to the increase in the use of artificial sweeteners. Remember, the typical consumer of diet beverages drinks an average of three a day. And researches and health experts are starting to ask whether it's possible that artificial sweeteners actually make us fatter? Are they raising, not lowering, the risk of diabetes? Could they actually be raising the risk of developing metabolic syndrome, often a precursor to cardiovascular disease?

Do a quick search on the Internet, and you will find medical experts and others who have voiced serious health concerns, saying that these sweeteners are toxic and might be associated with neurological issues, joint pain, vision problems, damage to the optic nerve, hair loss, migraines, dermatitis, and digestive and gastrointestinal problems, to name just a few. They point out that when we ingest aspartame (an ingredient in a majority of diet sodas), we are actually feeding our body formaldehyde. Consumers are currently ingesting one million pounds of aspartame per year. Is anyone actually suggesting that formaldehyde is good for anyone?

But focusing primarily here on the twin issues of fat and FAT*flammation*, medical experts also say that artificial sweeteners confuse our bodies, making them believe that sugar is forthcoming; this increases the production of insulin, which, in turn, makes our fat cells expand. (Think belly fat.) Researchers also point out that the original studies on the safety of artificial sweeteners were done years ago and may not have considered the degree to which they are now being consumed.

More recently, research has focused on whether or not artificial sweeteners contribute to our issues with fat, and the results are very disturbing:

▶ Studies show that artificial sweeteners can intensify "sweet" cravings, causing us to want sweeter and sweeter food, and lose our interest in nonsweetened food choices. This means that a normally sweet food such as an apple becomes less and less appealing; and vegetables have no appeal whatsoever.

▶ Animal studies show that artificial sweeteners are staggeringly addictive. When rats exposed to cocaine were given a choice between artificial sweeteners and cocaine, 94 percent of them chose the artificial sweetener.

▶ Human studies further show that artificial sweeteners encourage sugar cravings and sugar dependence.

▶ Several large-scale studies with human participants also show that there is a strong correlation between weight gain and artificial sweeteners. People who drank artificially sweetened soda were more likely to gain weight than those who drank nondiet soda.

▶ Other animal studies show that rats given artificial sweeteners actually ate more food. In fact, within a period of two weeks, the rats' metabolism slowed down and they gained a whopping 14 percent more body fat. In two weeks!

▶ A study of 66,118 women showed that artificially sweetened diet soda raised the risk of diabetes more than sugar-sweetened soda. Women who drank twelve ounces of diet soda a week had a 33 percent increased risk of type 2 diabetes, while women who consumed twenty ounces a week increased their risk by 66 percent.

► Studies also show that artificial sweeteners can reduce the number and balance of beneficial bacteria in the digestive tract. Increasing beneficial gut bacteria is an essential component in reversing FATflammation.

All the above studies show that artificial sweeteners, by tricking the brain and altering gut bacteria, lead to stronger cravings, deeper hunger, and continued fat storage—otherwise known as **FATflammation**.

Do you really need more convincing?

Are You Addicted to Artificial Sweeteners

Here is a quick quiz to help you determine whether you have an addiction to artificial sweeteners:

Are you using one or more packets of artificial sweetener daily to sweeten your coffee or tea?

When given a choice between real maple syrup and artificially sweetened maple syrup, do you choose the artificially sweetened version because you prefer the taste?

Do you drink at least one diet soda every day?

Do you actually like the taste of your preferred artificial sweetener?

Do you have a wide variety of artificially sweetened products (ketchup, gum, candy, cough drops) in your house?

Have any family members or friends expressed their concern about the number of diet sodas you are drinking?

Are you adding more and more artificial sweetener to your tea or coffee?

Are you failing to lose weight even though you have been using artificial sweeteners to replace sugar?

Are you losing your interest in natural foods (such as fruits and vegetables) because they are not sweet enough for your taste?

Even though you use artificial sweeteners, do you still have strong cravings for sugar and carbohydrate foods?

Have you read information telling you that diet sodas might be dangerous for your health and are you ignoring them because you don't want to stop drinking them?

If you answered yes to two or more of these questions, then you may well be addicted to artificial sweeteners.

I understand how hard it is to walk away from a bad relationship. You first have to recognize it's a bad relationship, then take the first step toward a healthier one. And there's no way around it: your relationship with the products and ingredients that cause FATflammation is so bad it's toxic. But the good news is it doesn't have to be like this. Although it may be painful and scary at first, you'll quickly find that after ridding yourself of the foods that inflame your fat cells and generally make you feel terrible about yourself, you'll start to feel—and look—better in almost no time at all.

CHAPTER 5

BURN FAT BY EATING (THE RIGHT) FAT

"Years ago, my husband read a book about dieting that said all fat was bad. He wouldn't even eat an avocado because the book said it was filled with fat. I went along with him and we only bought skim milk, fat-free yogurt and cheese, or sometimes, as a big treat, low fat. The only meat we eat is white meat chicken. Even so, I have weight problems. I don't understand it."

—MARIE

▶ Right now, in every supermarket in America, men and women are standing in front of the dairy section picking up containers of nonfat yogurt, filled with all kinds of sugared fruity syrup. These people honestly believe they are making less-fattening choices because the products they are bringing home are labeled "nonfat." They don't stop to read the labels telling them how much sugar and/or HFCS are in these products. All they can see is the slogan "0 fats."

Fat has received such a bad rap that many people are afraid of it. They live in downright terror of consuming it in any form. When a person with this kind of indoctrination looks at a nutrition label, he or she is interested in only two pieces of information:

1. What is the calorie count?

2. How many grams of fat?

For years, food consumers (that's all of us) have been brainwashed into believing that anything that is nonfat or low fat is healthy. We were given the wrong information by people who were themselves confused and didn't know or understand the facts. Better and more up-to-date research is now available, and we need to pay attention to it. A misunderstanding of calories and weight gain helped perpetrate the "all fat is bad" myth. Yes, fat typically has more calories than protein or carbohydrates, but that does not mean that it is, by definition, more "fattening." But that's what we were told to believe.

The "low-fat food will create weight loss" misinformation began back in the 1980s. Everyone heard the message. Food manufacturers absolutely know that most people today have a visceral reaction to the word *fat* and so you will see on food labels the words *Fat Free, Low-Fat, Lite or Light, Reduced Fat* and more. Many people, including some "health professionals" think that once someone starts eating foods that are low in fat, weight will drop off.

Not true.

Low-fat diets are one of the fastest ways to put on weight. Why? Because they leave us feeling hungry. Fat is very effective in sending a signal to the brain that says you are full. If you don't have enough fat in your diet, your body won't produce enough leptin to put the brakes on your hunger.

Similarly, low-fat diets are also frequently very low in protein. People on low-fat diets tend to avoid protein from animal sources because they contain saturated fat, forgetting that protein helps us lose weight. Food manufacturers who jumped on the "no-fat" bandwagon also removed as much fat from our food as possible. But when you remove fat from food, it also loses much of its taste. To compensate for this, manufacturers typically added ingredients like sugar and other refined carbohydrates, both of which are by definition inflammatory. *These* are the ingredients that have helped make us fat. In short, an incorrect understanding of fat has helped create a nation that is 68 percent overweight and filled with people struggling with FATflammation.

The truth is, our bodies need fat. Research shows that we indeed need fat to lose weight, stay healthy, and feel satiated. A sense of fullness, gained from the right foods, is one important key to weight loss.

Healthy fat will help you burn fat because it allows your body to respond more efficiently to leptin, the hormone that signals your body/brain to suppress your appetite.

People accustomed to hearing time and again "Don't eat fat!" now might have a difficult time believing "Eating fat burns fat!" But it's true. While there are without question fats that inflame fat cells, there are also a number of healthy fats that will—amazing—help you burn fat, as well as help you reduce inflammation. Once you start eating the right kind of essential fatty acids and start cutting back on the wrong kind, your fat cells will start to shrink, your FATflammation will begin to recede, and you will never fear fat again. Honest.

So which ones are the right fats, and which fats are the wrong ones?

OMEGA-3 FATS KEEP YOU THIN / OMEGA-6 FATS MAKE YOU FAT

Two essential fatty acids are necessary for our health and well-being: omega-3 and omega-6. They are called "essential" because we need them for our survival. The problem is that the body cannot produce them on its own. We can only get them from our diet. If you look at packaging on some food products today, you may notice something that informs you, the consumer, that the product is a source of omega-3 fatty acids. Packaging sometimes also informs consumers that the product contains ALA, alpha-linolenic acid, which is an omega-3 fatty acid.

The latest medical research confirms that both omega-3 and omega-6 are necessary for our well-being, but—and this is a huge BUT—we are in big trouble if we are not getting enough omega-3 in our diet and too much omega-6. That's because omega-3 reduces inflammation while excessive amounts of omega-6 increases it.

Take arachidonic acid, for instance. Arachidonic acid is an omega-6 fatty acid that's essential to life. Our bodies don't make it, and we need to get it from what we eat. But excessive amounts of arachidonic acid, which our bodies store in fat cells along with glucose and fat, will not only make us fat—it will also make us sick. When we have too much arachidonic acid, it causes damage to our fat cells, which leads to inflammation. Also, if the arachidonic acid sticks around or continues to circulate freely in our bodies, it will create inflammation throughout the body, causing a variety of health problems—definitely not what we want.

Common foods that contain high levels of omega-6 include corn, soybeans, and certain kinds of seeds, such as safflower and sunflower. Food manufacturers regularly include high concentrations of all these in popular vegetable and seed oils and, consequently, in salad dressings.

Conversely, omega-3 fish oil supplements, as well as foods rich in omega-3 fatty acids, such as cold water fish, can help lower your risk of a large number of health problems associated with inflammation, including arthritis, cancer, heart disease, and, even depression and other psychological issues. Omega-3 is also a great way to fight cellulite!

We are only now beginning to understand in full how too little omega-3 and too much omega-6 is making us fat. But we do know for certain that increasing the amount of omega-3 in your diet, while lowering the amount of omega-6, is one of the most important things you can do to fight FATflammation.

So now you're probably wondering, how much omega-3 do I need to eat? And how much omega-6 is too much?

Good Sources of Omega-3

Halibut	*Clams and mussels*
Herring	*Pasture-raised chickens (preferably*
Sardines	*organic)*
Wild-caught salmon	*Eggs from pasture raised chickens*
Tuna	*Pasture-raised meat (preferably organic)*
Lake trout	*Walnuts*
Mackerel	*Chia seeds*

When it comes to buying chickens and eggs, look for labels that read "pasture raised" as well as "organic." The term "pasture-raised" means that the chickens are spending most of their time in a pasture where they can forage for plants, seeds, and insects. The term "organic" tells you that even if the chickens' diet is supplemented by grains, those grains are GMO free.

Modern farming has altered the ways the animals you eat are raised. Until the 1940s cattle spent their days grazing on grasses, which is what they were meant to be eating. Cows and cattle are cud-chewing animals; they want to be out there munching on plants and grasses that are high in fiber. They were not meant to be kept in pens and feedlots eating high omega-6 corn- or soy-based diets, particularly GMO versions.

As Michael Pollan writes in *The Omnivore's Dilemma*, "You are what you eat is a truism hard to argue with, and yet it is, as a visit to a feedlot suggests, incomplete, for you are what what you eat eats, too. And what we are, or have become, is not just meat but number 2 corn and oil."

What's more, because these animals are being fed a diet that is not only wrong for them, but inflammatory, they, like humans, are getting sick; they are suffering from weakened immune systems as well as diarrhea, liver disease, ulcers, and digestive disorders. This means that they routinely require antibiotics. Some of the statistics I've seen indicate that about 70 to 80 percent of the antibiotics used in this country are being given to farm animals. This overuse of antibiotics is creating antibiotic-resistant bacteria. These bacteria are also found in the trillions of tons of animal waste created each year here in the United States. This could ultimately harm our natural ecosystems and threaten our water supply. So there are very serious health implications involved in what farm animals are eating.

For people trying to lose weight, there is another huge issue: cows that eat corn contribute to our problems with FATflammation. All that corn can't help but be inflammatory. In contrast, beef that comes from grass-fed cows naturally has a lower fat content, and the fat that is there is healthier for us to eat. Grass-fed cows have as much as 60 percent more omega-3 in their bodies; consequently, the ratio of omega -3 to omega-6 in their beef is much more favorable. Cows being fed a corn-based diet have a ratio of omega-3 to omega-6 that is somewhere in the neighborhood of 1:22. The ratio of omega-3 to omega-6 in grass-fed cows is about 1:2.

This FATflammation problem with corn-fed beef becomes even more problematic when the corn they are being fed is genetically modi-fied. One statistic that people who are opposed to genetically modified crops use to bolster their case: since GMO crops were introduced as feed, the incidence of people with three or more chronic diseases has nearly doubled, from 7 percent to 13 percent.

One of the best ways to buy eggs and fresh chicken is from a local farm or farmers' market where you can talk to the farmer or see for yourself how the chickens are raised.

Back in the day when our ancient ancestors were running around as hunter-gatherers, they were naturally eating food high in omega-3, at approximately a ratio of 1:1 to omega-6. The indigenous Inuit populations in the Arctic regions of Canada, Greenland, and the United States, for example, existed primarily on omega-3 seafood. In fact, they ate so much seafood, their ratio was an impressive 4:1 ratio. Other nonindustrial civilizations that ate mostly land animals had an omega-3/omega-6 ratio of approximately 1:3.

As civilization evolved, however, we have become more dependent on food manufacturing and factory farming, an unfortunate dependency that's dramatically jacked up the delicate ratio, which has gone up consistently over the past thirty years. The ideal ratio of omega-3/omega-6 is 1:1. However, a ratio of 1:4, which is still acceptable, would help keep us in a healthy range. Today, the typical ratio of omega-3 to omega-6 is approximately 1:16, but for some people the omega-6 in their diets is even higher. This imbalance between omega-3 and omega-6 fatty acids is, unfortunately, the norm. This imbalance has also helped create a nation of men and women with inflamed fat cells and a variety of acute and chronic illnesses, including obesity, diabetes, and heart disease.

What's happening? Sure, the average man or woman struggling with FAT-flammation is eating many fewer foods that are high in omega-3. Most of us are not eating enough fatty fish, and the meat and butter we do consume does not come from pasture raised animals. But the biggest reason behind this huge imbalance between omega-6 and omega-3 fatty acids is that we consume extraordinary amounts of foods high in omega-6 during every meal.

When I tell people to cut back on foods high in omega-6, they typically say something like, "But I'm not eating corn, peanuts, soybeans, or seeds. So what's the problem?" I always suggest they take a better look around their kitchens. Sure, they may not be eating whole food sources of omega-6, but few of us can avoid eating food products made *from* these sources. Canola oil, vegetable oil, and other popular cooking oils are predominantly made from sources of high omega-6, though they aren't necessarily labeled "high" in omega-6 fats. Becoming familiar with all the oil types high in omega-6 fats, and avoiding them, will markedly help to shrink your fat cells.

As an example, let's watch my friend, Jean, as she makes herself an egg for breakfast. Jean is trying very hard to lose weight so she avoids using butter because of the "fat." That's why, before breaking the egg, she puts a small amount of vegetable oil in a frying pan. She thinks the fact that the label says "Vegetable Oil" means that it is healthy. Jean then removes a piece of bread from a package labeled 100 percent whole wheat and tosses it into her toaster. Minutes later, she slathers on her toast a butter substitute from a container labeled "organic." She pours herself a cup of coffee and she sits down. It's a very simple meal.

But let's take a quick look at how much omega-6 is in her simple meal. Let's start with the vegetable oil. The label tells her that it's made from 100 percent soybean oil, which is incredibly high in omega-6. How about Jean's toast? Well, when we look at the package ingredients, we see that the bread includes, guess what? More soybean oil.

And what about the "organic" butter substitute? You guessed it. More soybean oil, along with crushed soybeans and soy lecithin—all of which are big sources of omega-6. So what's left in Jean's breakfast? Oh, yes, the egg. Jean is using an egg she purchased at the supermarket. It is not organic or from a pasture-raised chicken, which would create a higher ratio of omega-3. In fact, in all likelihood, it is coming from a chicken that was fed only corn and soybeans. That means that Jean's egg is also a source of omega-6. Without realizing it, Jean's simple meal could be directly contributing to her FATflammation.

Bottom line: omega-6 is ubiquitous. Even if we aren't getting it directly from our food choices, we are getting it indirectly because we are eating food like eggs, chicken, and meat pumped full of omega-6 grains, not to mention the double whammy of hormones and antibiotics.

Eicosanoids

We can't talk about balancing omega-3 and omega-6 fatty acids without discussing a group of hormones called "eicosanoids." Eicosanoids are derived from the essential omega-3 or omega-6 fatty acids provided by our diets. And, true to form, good eicosanoids are associated with omega-3, and bad eicosanoids are associated with omega-6.

Within the body, eicosanoids act as the ultimate messenger hormones. Working together to allow the cells to communicate with each other, eicosanoids strongly influence and even control many of our body's functions, including all forms of inflammation.

If you want to be healthy and fit, you need to keep your eicosanoids in balance. Barry Sears, Ph.D., a leading research scientist and author of *The Zone*, says, "It is the balance of eicosanoids in your body that is the ultimate key to wellness. Simply stated, the 'good' eicosanoids promote cellular rejuvenation; the 'bad' eicosanoids promote cellular destruction. You need both good and bad eicosanoids to survive. It's when the balance of these powerful hormones is disrupted and you start making too many bad eicosanoids that you begin moving away from wellness and toward the development of chronic disease." Once your cells begin to rejuvenate, not only will you start to feel better, you will look better.

SO MUCH SOY IS TOO MUCH SOY

No discussion of the amount of omega-6 in our diets is complete without mentioning soy and soy products, which we are all ingesting, often without realizing it. How did it happen? When did it happen? It wasn't that long ago that if you wanted to buy tofu, you had to visit a health food store. I remember the first time I had tofu. It was in a Chinese restaurant—tofu and Chinese vegetables. It was delicious, but definitely not something that I expected to eat regularly. It's amazing how quickly soy became such a popular product. One day, food made from soy seemed exotic and unusual; then, suddenly soy was everywhere.

The soy craze began for several reasons. Women, for example, were informed that soy was rich in phytoestrogens or isoflavones, which are plant hormones that can mimic estrogen. For women experiencing "hot flashes" and other menopausal symptoms, eating soy seemed to be an easy and natural way to replace estrogen. Vegetarians also made a quick leap onto the soy bandwagon because soy is a source of nonanimal protein. We were all told, and we believed that "soy is a health food."

Food manufacturers couldn't help but notice that people were buying more and more soy, and they quickly responded by creating and marketing more and more products featuring soy. Now, soy is in everything—soy ice cream, soy cheese, and soy milk. It's even easy to find soy hot dogs. In fact, just about all imitation meat products are filled with soy. When we eat tofu or drink soy milk, we know we are ingesting soy. But soy is also found in many, many products that we eat regularly without being aware of it. We find it in salad dressings, butter substitutes, oils used for cooking as well as for salads, and even bread. In short, everybody seems to be eating soy—lots of soy.

Here are some of the problems with soy:

You now know that omega-6 in excess creates FATflammation. Soy is very rich in omega-6 fatty acids.

Soy is also high in phytic acids, a compound that blocks the absorption of necessary minerals, most notably calcium, magnesium, and zinc, all of which are necessary for reduced inflammation and weight loss. Anyone concerned about osteoporosis or bone loss needs to think about calcium; anyone under stress needs to remember that low magnesium is often connected with an increase in stress-related symptoms. And zinc is associated with leptin, the hormone that helps reduce hunger.

As much as 90 percent of the soy produced in this country is genetically modified. GMO products have been linked to obesity and, as we know, much worse.

Soy disrupts your hormones. Because soy is a phytoestrogen, a plant-derived estrogen, it can have a significant effect on estrogen and testosterone levels, which, in turn, can impact a variety of health issues, including cancer. The research, which has often produced mixed results, is complicated and confusing at best. If you have questions about this, discuss it with your personal physician or medical practitioner.

Because soy is a goitrogen, it affects the function of the thyroid

gland and its uptake of iodine. There is some serious concern that ingesting large amounts of soy has a negative effect on the thyroid and might contribute to hypothyroidism. As we all know, thyroid issues are frequently associated with weight gain.

Soy increases your need for the very important nutrient vitamin D, because the phytic acid found in soy prevents adequate absorption.

FATflammation has one of its roots in digestive inflammation. Soy can create an inflamed digestive environment not just with inflamed fat cells, but also with digestive distress, such as bloating, diarrhea, constipation, gas, and heartburn.

Some people are very sensitive to soy. I had a client who came to me because she was chronically bloated. Like many people, she thought she was doing something good for her health by eating soy products. I suggested she remove soy from her diet for three days. The difference was remarkable. Her belly bloat went down, and her discomfort disappeared.

People who hear me talk about soy often have the same questions. They say, "Well Asians live longer than Americans and they eat a diet filled with soy. What's up with that?"

My answer: "The Asian diet mainly uses fermented soy such as miso, tempeh, and natto, not the processed junk soy Americans typically ingest. Also, they are using much smaller amounts of it. They aren't eating handfuls of edamame or soy nuts. They aren't chugging down glasses of processed soy milk daily and following it up with soy ice cream."

Soy is in many foods, and it can be sneaky, so read your ingredient labels and be on the lookout for foods that contain hidden and not so hidden soy. Here are some places we find soy.

Vegetable oil	Soy sauce
Soybean oil	Soy nuts
Hydrolyzed soy protein (HSP)	Soybeans
Soy lecithin	Soy milk
Soy protein	Textured vegetable protein

MELTING YOUR FAT WITH THE FAT YOU EAT

The bottom line on fat is very clear. You need healthy fats to help you burn off your fat. Eat the right omega-3 fats—and you will drop the weight. Eat too much of the wrong fats—omega-6 fats—and you'll store more fat. Because omega-6 is available in so many foods, it's almost impossible to avoid it altogether—nor should we. What we can do is avoid the manufactured foods that are particularly high in omega-6 such as corn oil and vegetable oil, both of which are made of soy. We can stop indulging in foods like corn chips and soy milk. When you eat out, make a point of asking what oils are being used for cooking. But one of the most important things you can do is increase your dietary intake of omega-3. The FATflammation-Free Diet Program includes a healthy fat with every meal and every snack. This will make a huge difference in helping you win your battle with FATflammation.

CHAPTER 6

BEAT SLUGGISH METABOLISM, FATFLAMMATION'S BFF

*"I love my friend Merilee, but I hate eating out with her.
She's five foot six and looks like she's a size 2, and she can
eat everything in sight without gaining an ounce. The last
time we ate out together, she had pasta Alfredo, polished
off the entire breadbasket, and for dessert she had some
kind of cream puff covered with chocolate sauce and
whipped cream. If I have even a bit of something she's
eating, I can feel the fat stuff landing on my hips."*

—KYLA

▶ Many of you reading this can probably identify with Kyla's experience. You probably understand what it means to struggle with a sluggish, slow-burning metabolism. You may also know what it feels like to have thin friends with high metabolism give you funny looks when you complain that you can't eat that much without gaining weight. People's reactions sometimes make you question your own experience. How is it possible, you ask yourself, for one person to be so quick to gain weight while another always seems to be eating?

"Is it possible," Kyla wonders, "that Merilee only eats when she is out socializing. Maybe Merilee is a secret dieter; maybe when she is home, she is on a starvation diet of celery stalks and bottled water. Maybe that's why she's so thin. How could our metabolism be so different?"

Here's a fact that we all need to acknowledge: sluggish metabolism is real.

Sluggish metabolism is FATflammation's troublemaking BFF. When it comes to getting rid of fat, "FatFlam" and "Sluggie" are two of the "meanest kids" in the playground of your life. They are almost always together, skipping around hand in hand, working as a team to keep you from achieving your weight-loss goals.

Each and every day, your body takes the food you eat and converts it into the energy you need to stay alive. The energy that is found in food is measured in terms of calories. Your metabolic rate describes the amount of energy (calories) your body uses to fulfill all its functions. If your metabolism stopped working, you would stop living. Without your metabolism, you wouldn't have enough energy for your heart to beat or any of your body's other systems to work. Every time you eat something, your metabolism jumps into action to keep your body doing what it needs to do.

Eating is necessary for survival. Your body needs a certain number of calories per day to keep your metabolism (and your life) going. If you go through days or even weeks or months in your life when you are eating less than that amount, your body gets very, very nervous. I repeat, *your body doesn't want you to starve*. It responds to extremely low calorie diets by slowing down your metabolism so you will need less food to survive. Repeated patterns of eating too little food can be as disastrous, in terms of eventual weight gain, as eating too much.

Perhaps even today you still have a very uneven eating pattern. Maybe you don't always eat breakfast or don't eat breakfast until you have been awake for hours. Perhaps you go all day without eating and then you spend the early evening making up for it. Maybe you often let yourself get so hungry that when you see food you want to eat everything in sight. All these patterns confuse your metabolism. Over a lifetime, these uneven patterns not only confuse your metabolism, they mess it up. A history of yo-yo dieting also contributes to muscle loss. If you have ever gone on a crash diet without establishing an exercise regime, the chances are that you lost more than fat. You also lost muscle. Then if you gain that weight back, it tends to return as fat. When your metabolism slows because of crash dieting and muscle loss, and you then go back to eating the way you normally did, you store more calories as fat. With each successive crash diet, your metabolism slows. That spells out weight gain.

We all burn up calories from the food we eat, but we all do it at a different rate. Numerous factors affect a person's metabolic rate, most notably age, genetics, gender, stress, and of course diet—not only what a person eats, but how they eat and how often. How often do you eat? Do you skip meals? Do you forget to eat breakfast? Do you eat late at night? All these habits make a difference in the rate at which our metabolism functions. At the same time, do you gulp down your food? Or do you chew at a leisurely pace? Yes, this makes a difference. Eating too quickly tends to slow down your metabolism, while eating at a leisurely pace speeds it up.

Do You Have Sluggish Metabolism?

If you have sluggish metabolism, you are probably all too aware of it. But here are some questions to help you assess your experience:

Do you have a very difficult time losing weight, no matter how much you diet or exercise?

Do you gain weight easily, no matter how much you restrict your diet?

Are you a woman over the age of thirty?

Are you a man over the age of forty?

Do you have strong cravings for sugar or carbohydrates particularly in the late afternoon or early evening?

Do you have a problem with dry skin?

If you are a woman, are you having hair loss?

Are you often under stress?

Do you sometimes forget to eat breakfast?

Do you sometimes go long periods without eating?

When you do eat, however, do you tend to eat more than you should?

Is protein often noticeably absent from your meals and/or snacks?

Was there ever a time in your life when you exercised a great deal and ate very little?

Do you have a history of yo-yo dieting?

Do you have a problem with cellulite?

If you answered yes to more than four of the above questions, then you probably have "sluggish metabolism."

When we use the term "metabolism," we are usually describing basal or resting metabolism. Even if you did nothing but sleep and rest all day long, your basal (or resting) metabolism is still doing what it has to do to keep you alive and your body systems working. Simply staying alive requires approximately 70 percent of the energy your body expends. Another 20 percent is spent on movement or physical activity. The remaining 10 percent is used for digestion and processing the food you eat.

HOW YOUR BODY UTILIZES THE FOOD YOU EAT	
Calories expended (burned up) from basal metabolism	70 percent
Calories expended (burned up) by physical movement	20 percent
Calories expended (burned up) by the process of digesting food	10 percent

In addition to simply staying alive and exercising, there are other efficient ways to help speed up a sluggish metabolism. One of the easiest ways to speed up your metabolism and burn fat in the process is by adding more protein to your diet.

Protein is made up of building blocks known as amino acids. There are approximately twenty different amino acids that come together to make up all different kinds of protein. Some of these amino acids, like fatty acids, are "essential amino acids," which as you'll recall means we need to get them from our food because the body can't produce them on its own. Amino acids are necessary for life; once converted by the body, they "feed" all of our tissues, cells, and organs. If our diets don't provide enough protein, we are lacking in the building blocks that keep us alive.

In addition to keeping you alive and kicking, protein helps boosts your metabolism, just as omega-3 fats do. This is not a myth or an urban legend. It's true: your body burns more calories in the process of digesting protein than it does digesting carbohydrates or fats. Think about that for a second. *Protein helps your body burn more calories than carbs or fats.*

I always tell clients to include protein with every meal and snack because it will boost their metabolism. Many love this advice; others start out with significantly less enthusiasm. Some people always tend to gravitate toward carbohydrates. Sometimes, even in the very best steak restaurants, people order mac and cheese and creamed spinach. Or, at home, they tend to specialize in high-carbohydrate meals; for snacks, they focus on sugar-filled treats or foods that crunch—crackers, potato chips, and popcorn. It's sometimes difficult for them to become accustomed to the idea of including more protein. But if you are really serious about losing weight and winning your fight against FATflammation, you have to get serious about eating protein.

In fact, I never cease to be amazed at how quickly protein can make a difference in someone's life. I remember one of my clients, Chris. When he started working with me, Chris weighed close to four hundred pounds, a weight he'd carried for about twenty years. Chris was a very dynamic person and he was accustomed to achieving his goals. He had heard all those messages about high-carbohydrate/low-fat diets being healthy; he had paid attention and tried to eat accordingly. Chris typically started his day with cereal and a glass of orange juice. His other favorite breakfast was a large container of fruit salad and toast. When he arrived at work, he might have some donuts or a few packages of crackers and cheese. Sometimes he had a bagel.

For lunch, Chris would usually have a sandwich with some kind of deli meat, on a big crunchy French roll along with a bag of chips. Throughout the day, he continually drank soda, his drink of choice. If there were any cookies or cake available, Chris didn't hesitate. Chris also loved to snack on fruit, particularly bananas, which he ate daily. He also liked mangoes and pineapple.

He definitely went overboard with the fruit. Chris thought fruit was a very healthy choice.

For dinner, Chris would most often make himself a very large bowl of pasta. Because he wanted to be healthy, he sometimes chose a whole wheat or whole-grain pasta with a tomato-based sauce. After dinner, he had dessert—something like frozen yogurt. And he frequently also ate more fruit.

Looking at Chris's diet, the obvious question to ask is: Where is the protein? It wasn't there. One of the first things I asked Chris to do was to have six ounces of protein with every meal and to include protein with every snack. He also started taking an omega-3 fish oil supplement and added some healthy fats such as olive oil, avocado, and nuts. And he reduced his consumption of carbohydrates, including the fruit. I told Chris he could have as many veggies as he wanted. In my experience, men are more likely to gravitate toward protein-filled foods, and Chris found it relatively painless to start including more protein. Eventually Chris lost about two hundred pounds. Yes, Chris had been eating a great deal of food, but he was often hungry because he was eating very little protein. I really do believe that the inclusion of more protein in his diet gave him the push he needed.

Protein definitely makes you feel satisfied and satiated. Many of us have had the experience of "downing" a huge carbohydrate-filled meal and then feeling hungry within a short time. That's not what happens when we eat protein, regardless of its source, whether it's from an animal or a plant. Protein makes us feel fuller and it happens faster. After high-protein meals, we are less likely to feel as though we want more food, because protein triggers hormones that tell your body that you have had enough to eat. That's why dieters who include protein with all their meals tend to feel less deprived than those who don't. Recent studies indicate that eating a high-protein breakfast will help curb your appetite and decrease cravings for carbohydrates such as sugar throughout the day and even into the evening. Eating two eggs for breakfast, for example, puts the brakes on both hunger and cravings for hours longer than a carbohydrate-centered breakfast.

Similarly, protein stimulates the release of glucagon, a hormone produced within the pancreas. While insulin lowers glucose when it gets too high, glucagon raises it when it gets too low, which means insulin and glucagon work in tandem to keep our blood sugar stable. Glucagon also helps burn up stored fat from our fat cells.

Protein also helps build muscle—and the more muscle you have, the more calories you burn. But don't get confused: even though protein helps with muscle synthesis (the muscle-building process), you're not going to get the muscle or tone you want without exercise.

Boosting Your Metabolism

Here are some tips that will help you fight FATflammation, as well as boost your metabolism.

Have Your Thyroid Hormone Levels Checked

I always suggest that anyone starting a diet plan get a thorough medical checkup that includes a blood test to check the level of your thyroid hormones. Low thyroid output is a very common (and often hidden) cause of weight gain.

Stay Well Hydrated

As soon as you wake up each morning, drink eight ounces of water. Then drink two eight-ounce glasses of cool water before breakfast, lunch, and dinner. There is research showing that drinking two glasses of cool water before each of your meals will boost your resting metabolism enough to lose five pounds a year, even if you do nothing else.

Don't Forget Your Protein

Make certain every meal *and* every snack includes a good source of protein because it will give your metabolism an additional boost. Remember, the protein you eat doesn't have to be meat. A piece of celery filled with a tablespoon of peanut butter, for example, includes fiber, a complex carb, and, yes, protein.

Always Eat Breakfast

Have breakfast soon after you wake up—within thirty minutes. Eating breakfast reminds your metabolism to kick into gear. Studies also show that those who eat breakfast lose more weight and have an easier time keeping the weight off than those who do not.

Eat Regularly

I recommend three meals a day and two snacks. This helps keep the metabolism humming and helps avoid hunger and cravings.

Practice Slower Eating

When you are eating, take your time and chew slowly. Your metabolism speeds up when you eat slow and slows down when you eat fast.

Add Some Heat to What You Eat

Capsaicin, which is found in peppers such as chili, habanero, and jalapeño, gives your metabolism a temporary boost. The same thing is true of ginger, black pepper, and hot mustard. This is a good tip for people who have an easy time digesting spicy food.

Don't Eat Late at Night

Eating when you should be sleeping stops the natural fat burn (ketosis) that takes place during the night.

Keep Moving

Don't sit still for long periods of time. Even if you have a desk job, make a point of moving around as much as you can. Move your arms and legs while you are sitting in a chair. Get up every thirty minutes. I like to do ten squats, which takes roughly ten seconds, but if you have trouble with squats, do ten leg lifts on each side. If there is a water cooler, walk out and get some water. Walk around your desk and stretch. When you get home, don't collapse into a chair or couch and stay there without budging. Do as much walking as you possibly can. Swing your arms as you go through life. Even fidgeting makes a difference in how you burn those calories. There is actually interesting research about the weight-loss benefits enjoyed by people who fidget.

Take Control of the Stress in Your Life

Stress bumps up your cortisol, which, in turn, slows down your metabolism, which increases your fat. When stressed, many of us also reach for food. Find a form of relaxation that works for you. This is very important.

Exercise Smart

There is a section later in this book about high-intensity interval training. I'm a big believer in this approach to exercise because it has worked for me and my clients. This form of exercise significantly cuts down the amount of time you need to spend exercising. High-intensity interval training really boosts your metabolism and helps you fire up your fat burn! Whatever you do, you need to find an exercise program that works for you. Many people like riding their bikes on bike paths throughout the country. I know several men and women who swim or do water aerobics. This can be as calming as it is healthful.

Add Some Green Tea to Your Life

A human study has shown that green tea boosts the metabolic rate and promotes fat oxidation, also known as "fat burn."

Have a Cup of Coffee or Black Tea

Research shows that both coffee and tea help boost metabolism. You don't want to drink so much that you're feeling "wired" or stressed because this could trigger cortisol. But a little bit of caffeine will go a long way toward helping your metabolism.

Take Your Vitamin D$_3$

Simply put, vitamin D$_3$ helps with muscle function and keeping your insulin levels healthy. Some research shows that people who are overweight are also more likely to be deficient in vitamin D. Animal studies have shown that vitamin D$_3$ results in an increase in lean mass. Human studies indicate that people with higher serum D$_3$ levels have a decreased risk for falls and muscle weakness as well as less insulin resistance and diabetes. People are not always informed about their vitamin D$_3$ levels. If you have blood work done, you need to request that the test for vitamin D$_3$ is included. Many of my clients—including some medical professionals—have started out with low levels of vitamin D$_3$. Once they began to take it regularly, they saw a marked effect in their weight and their health.

Watch Out for Pesticides

Research shows that pollutants from pesticides can be stored in your fat cells; this can cause a dip in your metabolism. There is also some interesting research indicating that pesticides are implicated in weight gain. Whenever possible, buy organic produce. Whether it's organic or conventional, wash your fruits and vegetables very, very carefully.

WHAT KIND OF PROTEIN SHOULD YOU EAT TO BEAT FATFLAMMATION?

Start by looking for proteins that are high in omega-3 fatty acids. Fish is always a good choice. Fresh wild salmon or canned wild salmon are particularly high in omega-3. Other fish choices high in omega-3 fatty acids include tuna, cod, sardines, anchovies, and mussels. Most seafood is desirable on the FATflammation-Free Diet Program.

Poultry and beef are also good sources of protein. Farm-raised grass-fed beef is always preferable because it has a better ratio of omega-3 to omega-6 oils. For both poultry and beef, organic is always better than nonorganic because in all likelihood organically raised animals are not getting GMO feed.

Dairy is a good protein choice. Milk from grass-fed cows will have higher omega-3 content and is always preferable. Choose milk that has a 1 or 2 percent fat content.

And don't forget nonanimal sources of protein. Beans and lentils and other legumes are particularly high in protein. Nuts and nut butters contain both healthy fats and protein, but be careful. If you are buying nut butters, read the labels. Don't buy anything with added sugar or hydrogenated oils. Almonds and walnuts are good choices, and some seeds are also great sources of protein. Sunflower seeds, in particular, contain a fair amount of protein, though you'll notice that sunflower oil is not allowed on the FATflammation-Free Diet Program because it is so high in omega-6. Other seeds like hemp, flax, and chia are also high in omega-3.

Because the FATflammation-Free Diet Program stresses increasing omega-3 fatty acids while reducing omega-6, I only suggest fermented soy products like tempeh and natto.

You can also find protein in unexpected places. For example, occasionally, try adding some quinoa, a nutrient-dense grain to your diet.

HOW MUCH PROTEIN SHOULD YOU BE EATING

I don't want you to think that I am advocating a primarily protein-centered diet with minimal carbohydrates, like the Atkins diet. Nothing could be further from the truth. Yes, you can initially lose weight on very high-protein, low-carbohydrate diets, but they are difficult to sustain and can ultimately increase inflammation because of the increase in arachidonic acid. Diets that are low in fiber are also bad for the health of your gut, and if you want to stay FATflammation free, you need a healthy gut.

Revving Up Metabolism with Protein Powders

WHEY POWDER

Whey is a by-product of cheese made from cow's milk; it's very popular among body builders and other athletes, because it helps build lean muscle, especially when combined with exercise. And the more muscle you have, the more calories you burn, which leads to greater weight loss. If you are putting on some weight as you get older, you are not alone. As we age, starting in our late twenties, we naturally also begin to lose muscle. If you have FATflammation and are experiencing a natural loss in muscle, this is a prescription for weight gain. If you follow the FATflammation-Free Diet Program and are also able to add more muscle mass to your body, you should start seeing marked changes. I've personally witnessed an increase in muscle mass and a reduction of fat in clients who have added an effective quality protein such as whey to their diets.

Whey also helps reduce appetite. Remember CCK? Whey helps stimulate this appetite-reducing hormone, and it may also increase levels of glutathione in the body. Glutathione, you may remember, functions as both an antioxidant and anti-inflammatory.

There are three major types of whey: whey protein concentrate (WPC), whey protein isolate (WPI), and whey protein hydrolysate. The type I use and suggest to others is the protein isolate, which is typically processed to be lower in fat and lactose. It's approximately 90 percent lactose free.

PEA-RICE POWDER

This is a good protein powder choice for vegetarians/vegans or the lactose intolerant. Pea-rice protein is gluten free and is comparable to whey in its positive health benefits. Like whey, it will help synthesize muscle, aid in muscle recovery, and balance blood sugar. It also slows production of the hormone ghrelin, which provides a thermic effect for weight loss.

There are several other protein powders, including hemp powder, brown rice powder, and pea powder. All of these can be added to food such as smoothies, yogurt, or oatmeal to put additional protein in your diet.

I recommend that every time you have something to eat, whether it's a meal or a snack, include some protein. How much? A good dinner or lunch portion of protein is about four to six ounces. That should measure about the size and thickness of the palm of your hand—similar in size to a deck of cards. A snack-size portion of dairy protein should be approximately half a cup of yogurt or cottage cheese. If you are eating nuts as a snack, figure on about eight nuts, or about one tablespoon of nut butter. If you are eating chicken, roast beef, or turkey as part of a snack, think in terms of one to two deli slices, depending on the thickness of the slice.

Because protein boosts your metabolism, a source of protein is included with every meal and snack in the FATflammation-Free Diet Program.

CHAPTER 7

BE KIND TO BUGS

*"The bacterial makeup of the intestines may help
determine whether people gain weight or lose it . . ."*
—FROM: "BACTERIA IN THE INTESTINES MAY HELP TIP THE
BATHROOM SCALE, STUDIES SHOW," *NEW YORK TIMES*, MARCH 27, 2013

▶ One of the secret ways to beat FATflammation is maintaining a healthy gut filled with healthy "bugs." Recent research shows that digestive flora, and the health of the digestive tract in general, plays a significant role in weight gain. I've certainly seen this in my own clients. An unhealthy digestive tract is an inflamed digestive tract. If you have an inflamed digestive tract, there's a good chance that you will also have inflamed fat cells—and vice versa.

Frequently, men and women with weight issues are concurrently struggling with gastrointestinal issues. They complain of regular bouts of indigestion and unreliable bowel patterns; they say that they are suffering from acid reflux, constipation, and irritable bowel syndrome. They spend large amounts of money at the drugstore buying a variety of over-the-counter medications including Pepcid, Prilosec, Prevacid, Zantac, Gasex, Immodium, as well as the old reliables like Pepto-Bismol, Milanta, Maalox, and Tums. Because they want to be smart about their health, they sometimes have endoscopies and colonoscopies. But these tests often don't show anything that fully explains their symptoms. It's incredibly frustrating to walk around with a series of uncomfortable gastrointestinal complaints and not know what to do next.

THE HUMAN MICROBIOME—
THE "FORGOTTEN ORGAN"

Before you reach for your own personal favorite digestive remedy, here are some things you need to know.

Your body provides a "comfy home" for trillions and trillions of microorganisms or microbes. It's estimated that there are ten times as many microbes in your body as there are human cells. Each of these microorganisms is so incredibly small that if you were able to put all of them together, they would make up between 1 and 3 percent of your total body mass. The community of all these microorganisms is called the human microbiome. And guess what? A large number of these microbiota live in your digestive system. Whether you call them bacteria, microorganisms, or microbes, these are the good and bad bugs in your gut. And, whether you like it or not, they are part of you, sharing your space. But they are not all the same; in fact, there are literally hundreds of different species.

We often tend to assume that anything labeled "microbe" or "bacteria" has, by definition, a negative role in your life. But that's not the case. In fact, most of these minuscule microbiota perform a positive function and help keep us healthy. Some of them help us digest carbohydrates, for example; others help make use of vitamins. We have often heard the "friendly" microbes that live in your digestive system referred to as "gut flora," "microflora," or just plain "flora." Some researchers describe the entire community of all the microbiota in our bodies as "the forgotten organ."

WHAT'S THE CONNECTION BETWEEN YOUR
MICROBIOME AND INFLAMMATION?

"You are what you eat, and so are the bacteria that live in your gut."
—"The Gut's Microbiome Changes Rapidly with Diet," *Scientific American*

The fat cells in your body and many of the microorganisms in your digestive system have similarly negative responses to sugar, processed grains, and junk foods. You know by now that sugar-filled and processed low-nutrient foods make our fat cells get fatter. What you may not know is that poor diets encourage and allow the more treacherous microbes in our bodies to flourish while simultaneously reducing the number of friendlier bacteria. Sugar feeds the bad gut bacteria, promoting even more FATflammation. It's not surprising that the standard American diet, SAD for short, can negatively alter the makeup of the complex ecosystem known as our microbiome, causing it to turn into a more hostile environment.

Your diet holds a great deal of responsibility for your digestive flora—the kind of microbes that are running around in your digestive system. A recent study indicates that the microbes in your gut start responding very rapidly—within days—to changes in your diet. Improve the quality of the food you eat, and you immediately alter the makeup of your microbiome, sometimes overnight. This is an important piece of information for anyone who is interested in getting healthier and losing weight.

But like fingerprints, no two people have the same microbiome.

The community of microbes in your body is always in flux depending upon your environment, what you eat, and your exposure to other bacteria. We come into the world with no microbiota in our systems. That changes immediately because our bodies are colonized by bacteria from our mothers—breast milk being one example. Even as we are being born, we start taking on microbes from our mothers. Interestingly, it would appear that infants who are born by cesarean birth don't receive some important microbes from their mothers. In fact, research shows that C-section children are twice as likely to become obese as children who experience normal birth. There is some speculation that the reason for this is that infants born by C-section have a different composition of bacteria than those who enter life through the birth canal. Both childhood obesity and C-section births have risen dramatically over the last few decades. During this time, there has also been also an increased risk for allergies and asthma in children, particularly those who have had a C-section or surgical delivery.

By the time we become adults, we have grown our own special group of microbes. They are the result of our environment, our food, how we live, the toxins and microbes to which we've been exposed, and the antibiotics we have taken.

Stop and think about what it is that antibiotics are designed to do. Antibiotics kill the microbes, both bad and good, living within our bodies. When antibiotics do their job, by definition, it means that these medications are changing the microbiome—the community of bacteria that live inside our bodies. When we take prescribed antibiotics, we lose harmful bacteria, but we also lose helpful bacteria.

Many scientists are currently asking whether the obesity epidemic in this country could be caused by the increase in antibiotic use. Most of us have received antibiotics. There is no denying their importance and value. But there is also no way around the fact that all those antibiotics have changed, perhaps permanently, our individual microbiomes. We know that antibiotics are miracle drugs that have saved lives. But are they also making us fat, just as they have helped fatten up the livestock we eat?

Your microbiome is incredibly complex, and science still doesn't know enough about how the "good" bacteria and the "more problematic" bacteria interact and impact your health and well-being. We don't understand, for example, how some bacteria have both "bad" and "good" qualities. This is a subject that can have important implications. For a moment, let's talk about *Heliciobacter pylori* (*H. pylori*), a specific bacteria about which we know a few things. Until the mid-1980s, it was pretty much universally believed that stomach ulcers were caused by stress and diet. Then some scientists saw the association between *H. pylori* bacteria found within our bodies and ulcers. It turned out that instead of being a stress-induced ailment, ulcers were caused by *H. pylori*! Eureka! This was a major breakthrough. Ulcers were quickly recognized as a treatable bacterial infection. In the last twenty years, most men and women suffering from ulcers have been receiving antibiotic treatment. This has made an amazing difference in the lives of many people. They have been protected from peptic ulcers as well as some types of cancer. But . . . nothing is that simple.

One of the most common antibiotics used to treat *H. pylori* is amoxicillin, which as we know, is often prescribed for a great many other infections. Both children and adults are regularly given amoxicillin. The end result is that this once common bacteria has been killed off in many people by antibiotic use. But now, we have a problem because it would appear that *H. pylori* has both good and bad roles within our bodies. There is evidence, for example, that *H. pylori* gives us some protection against asthma and allergies.

But what does that have to do with weight gain?

As amazing as it may seem, it turns out that *H. pylori* also has a working relationship with two hormones connected to weight gain. Ghrelin, a hormone that increases our appetite and makes us hungry, and leptin, the hormone that tells us that we are full. Then newest research tells us that when colonies of *H. pylori* are hanging out in your body, your ghrelin levels go down. As *H. pylori* in your body is eradicated and disappears, your ghrelin levels go up. In other words, you become hungrier and want more food. Is that your stomach growling?

Unfortunately, when *H. pylori* levels are reduced, the leptin in our bodies goes down as well. In short, as *H. pylori* disappears, we are also losing an important check that tells us to stop eating. This can make a significant difference for people, including children, who have been given large doses of antibiotics.

Keeping the bacteria in your gut happy is one of the best things you can do to reverse FATflammation and stay healthy. There are two easy ways to help you do this.

Make Probiotics Part of Your Life

Probiotics are helpful bacteria that help us maintain and restore the natural balance of flora in the digestive tract. Yogurt, a fermented milk product that contains cultures of helpful bacteria, is the probiotic most of us know best. Yogurt is an ancient food. It's even mentioned in the Old Testament; apparently, yogurt with honey was a "big treat" even then. Currently, the yogurt section of our local supermarkets is huge, with dozens of varieties being sold. But it wasn't that many years ago that if you wanted a container of yogurt, you had to make a trip to a health food store. It also wasn't that long ago that many M.D.s made fun of what they sometimes referred to as health food "nuts" who promoted foods like yogurt. That's changed. These days most doctors are routinely advising their patients to eat yogurt whenever they are taking prescribed antibiotics. Be sure to buy yogurts that say that the manufacturer is using live and active cultures. Many yogurts today are also filled with sugar, which, unfortunately, is turning our favorite health food into one of our favorite junk foods; they may contain as much sugar as a candy bar. Walk away from any yogurt that has added sugar or HFCS listed on the ingredient label.

Other cultured foods that contain probiotics include sauerkraut, kimchi, kefir, miso, and some cheeses like Gouda.

You can also buy probiotic supplements and take them daily. (Probiotics are included in the protocol to reverse FATflammation.)

Some interesting studies have been done with mice indicating that probiotics can help us get rid of fat. In one recent study, for example, researchers were able to make mice thinner or fatter by changing their gut bacteria. Another study done in Europe showed that lean people had higher microbial diversity than those who were more obese. Perhaps the most interesting research was done in Canada. For that study, 125 obese men and women were split into two groups for twenty-four weeks. During this period, one-half the subjects received two pills each day that contained probiotics from the Lactobacillus rhamnosus family. During the first twelve, all the men and women received the same kind of supervised, calorie-specific diet program. For the second twelve weeks, although each of the participants continued with a diet plan, calorie restrictions were lifted.

When the first twelve-week period ended, women who were taking the probiotics lost an average of 9.7 pounds. The women who weren't getting any probiotics had an average weight loss of 5.7 pounds. During the second twelve-week period, results become even more impressive. The women who were not taking probiotics were able to maintain their weight, but there was no further weight loss. The women taking probiotics, however, continued to lose weight. By the time the study was finished, the women taking probiotics lost approximately twice as much weight as the women who were not.

Make Prebiotics a Part of Your Life

Prebiotics is the catchall name we use when describing certain carbohydrates, known as nondigestible oligosaccharides. The foods in this category are not digested until they reach the large intestine, which is where they undergo fermentation. Prebiotics are beneficial because they help the friendly bacteria in your digestive system flourish and stay in control. Prebiotics are helpful to our gut because they contain "inulins," which are a class of dietary fibers. Inulin, for example, has been shown to selectively stimulate the growth of *Bifidobacteria* and *Lactobacillus,* two very beneficial bacteria. Including prebiotics in our diets also help boost the beneficial action of probiotics such as yogurt.

Prebiotic foods containing inulin include:

Dandelion greens	**Oatmeal**
Garlic	**Maple syrup**
Leek	**Jerusalem artichoke**
Onion	**Wheat bran**
Asparagus	**Yacon**
Chicory root	

Take a look at that list. You can't help but notice that many of the foods on it have long and established histories of promoting good health. For most of us, these are good foods to include in our diets. There are, of course, some people who are sensitive to dietary fiber. They complain of side effects such as bloating, gas, cramping, and diarrhea. So if you're not accustomed to eating these foods regularly, try them a little at a time and see how you react.

There are also several supplements that include inulin. These supplements are typically marketed as prebiotics. Chicory root is often an important ingredient. Lately we've been hearing more about weight reduction connected to yacon syrup, a natural sweetener that comes from yacon, a plant grown in the Andes. Yacon is also a prebiotic and includes inulin.

Your Gut and Your Emotional and Mental Well-Being

Many of us have always intuitively believed that a connection exists between the state of our emotions and our gastrointestinal systems. We know that when we are upset and stressed, we may also have problems with our digestion. Large numbers of us have seen firsthand that anxiety can bring on indigestion or bouts of diarrhea. We've probably also seen it work the other way and have become more nervous, anxious, or stressed after eating certain foods. Some people even believe there is a connection between depression and the foods we eat. Scientists are now asking whether there is a connection between the bacteria in our digestive system and our brain chemistry. In one study with mice, for example, stress led to memory problems. Yet, when the mice were given probiotics, that memory dysfunction disappeared, even in the presence of continued stress. It would appear that there's a direct line of communication between the gut and the brain via the vagus nerve. It's like having a direct line to the president of the United States from a special red phone. Isn't that cool?

FATFLAMMATION AND YOUR DIGESTIVE SYSTEM

It seems apparent that the health of your gut can lead to the health of your overall system, which means NO FATflammation! Wow! We really are what we eat. It's definitely time to move away from diets and lifestyles that can harm your gut. It's not too late to make the necessary change to claim your digestive health. Here are some "gut-healthy" suggestions to help you do this.

Start eating more foods that are higher in prebiotic, soluble fiber.

Eliminate the external toxins that can harm your digestive system. (Buy organic fruits and vegetables as much as possible and wash all fruits and vegetables well.)

Stop eating processed, refined foods.

Supplement your diet with probiotic foods, paying particular attention to fermented foods.

Take a probiotic supplement.

Try eating a Granny Smith apple a day. Scientists at Washington State University recently did a study that showed eating a Granny Smith apple a day could change the flora in your gut, causing it to behave more like that of a thin person, with fewer cravings and less hunger. The study also showed that Granny Smiths, specifically, contain high amounts of a fat-busting fiber called "pectin" that can keep you feeling satiated for hours.

Start exercising. A recent study from University College Cork showed that athletes have more beneficial bacteria in their guts than nonathletes. So start moving.

CHAPTER 8

BEWARE THE BANE OF GRAIN

" 'Eat more healthy whole grains' is among the biggest health blunders ever made in the history of nutritional advice."
—Dr. William Davis, author of *Wheat Belly*

▶ By now, we know that the refined grains we find in white bread, pretzels, cereal, white rice, pasta, macaroni, crackers contribute to FATflammation. But what about whole grains? For years, we had been told that whole grains are an important part of a healthy diet. Whole grains are filled with fiber. Don't we need more fiber in our diets? But now, some experts are saying things like "Wait just a minute, put down that bread." So what's the story with grains? We've received so much confusing advice. As a category, grains are food crops grown for their seeds, which are then ground to make flour, which sounds harmless enough. But the question remains, are grains good for us or is there something about grains—even those grains that we think of as healthy—that can make our fat cells grow even fatter? Well, it's complicated.

LET'S START WITH WHEAT

Until about ten thousand years ago, wheat and other grain products were not part of the human diet. Early hunter-gatherers didn't know how to grind wheat or bake bread. Even now, when we are further along in our evolutionary development, some people question whether our bodies are really equipped to process wheat in a healthful way. It's a serious question: Is the human body designed to eat wheat products? Recently several very persuasive and successful books say no and advise us all to give up wheat. And many people—from movie stars to the guy next door—have decided to do just that. Why are so many people giving up wheat?

Several issues are involved with eating wheat. Let's start by saying that it contains gluten, a protein. Other grains, such as barley and rye, also contain gluten. Some people are gluten intolerant. The most extreme form of gluten intolerance is celiac disease, which affects approximately three million Americans. People with celiac disease are unable to digest gluten and have a severe reaction to all wheat products; gluten triggers an immune response that is damaging to their intestinal tract.

Many other men and women suffer from the much milder, but still unpleasant and uncomfortable, gluten intolerances, all of which are contributory causes of FATflammation. If you are gluten intolerant, your fat cells will become even more irritated and inflamed if you eat anything containing gluten. Common symptoms of gluten intolerance include bloating, gas, and diarrhea, and other irritating digestive problems. Some people also feel tired, dizzy, or light-headed after eating gluten-laced products, while others suffer from headaches or dermatological problems. I had one client whose gluten sensitivity appeared to rear its ugly head in the form of cellulite. Once we removed all gluten from her diet, her cellulite amazingly vanished.

How do you know if you have gluten intolerance? The easiest way is to remove all gluten from your diet for a week. If you start to feel better, gluten may be your issue. Wait a couple of weeks and then eat some bread or pasta. How do you feel? If you start feeling crummy, you're most likely gluten intolerant. If you think you may be gluten intolerant, start reading food labels with great care because gluten can be found in a huge number of food products, ranging from artificial food colors to soy sauce and veggie burgers. Look for the following words on an ingredient label: *wheat, rye, wheatberries, farina, graham, kamut, einkorn, semolina, barley, wheat starch, seitan,* and *bulgur.* If you are highly sensitive to gluten, you also need to avoid oats processed in facilities that process other foods with gluten.

Most of us, though, aren't gluten intolerant. We can eat wheat in moderation without experiencing any acute external or internal sensitivities or any major autoimmune complications. But that doesn't mean we're entirely in the clear. The problem with wheat is bigger than gluten, particularly when it comes to FATflammation. Remember how refined grains—one of the FATflammation Four—causes inflammation because our bodies metabolize processed grains like sugar? Well, our bodies can often process wheat in a similar way—even though wheat, in its natural form, is a whole food. But the wheat we're eating today is far from its natural form. "This thing being sold to us called wheat," according to William Davis, M.D., the author of the bestselling *Wheat Belly,* "it ain't wheat. It's this stocky little high-yield plant, a distant relative of the wheat our mothers used to bake muffins, genetically and biochemically light years removed from the wheat of just 40 years ago."

Modern wheat is simply more inflammatory. I realize that it doesn't seem fair that bread and pasta, two foods that are so ubiquitous in our culture and society should cause FATflammation. But they do. And our modern wheat supply is heavily implicated in this situation. For thousands and thousands of years, humans cultivated and ate wheat without getting fat. Then in the last hundred years, technology changed the methods that had been working for all those years. It's all different: wheat, even whole wheat, is now grown, processed, and prepared differently; the seeds that are being grown are genetically and biologically different. The ancient varieties of wheat that were commonly used have been replaced by high-yield dwarf wheat that is less expensive to grow. Modern wheat is considered a "supercarbohydrate," and it has a more dramatic effect on blood glucose levels than the ancient grains, triggering insulin and increasing FATflammation.

However, I understand the problems involved in completely doing away with all wheat products. Assuming you are not gluten sensitive, the FATflammation-Free Diet Program allows for small amounts of whole wheat. **Ideally, the bread and pasta you eat should be sprouted and/or made from ancient grains such as einkorn.** Fortunately it's becoming easier to find these grains, which have the additional advantage of containing less gluten. When shopping for products containing einkorn, look on the label for the term "whole einkorn wheat." Sprouted grains will most likely be announced on the front of the package, or listed in the ingredients as "sprouted whole wheat." Some supermarkets keep these breads in their freezers, in order to keep them fresh. The lack of additives or chemicals limits a bread's shelf life, but as I'm sure you understand by now, increases our health and longevity.

WHAT ABOUT CORN?

Raise your hand if you thought corn was a vegetable. Well, it's not. It starts out as a grain. Whether you realize it or not, corn is found in all kinds of foods—corn flour, cornmeal, corn oil—and it's all inflammatory. It's also the food that is most likely to be genetically modified, which makes it even more inflammatory. These days, genetically modified sweet corn is everywhere, including your supermarket and local farm stands. Organic farmers are not allowed to use genetically modified seed in organic corn. If you care about not eating GMO products, as I do, the only safe place to buy your summer corn is from an organic grower or a local farmer, who knows what he/she is doing and is completely honest about what is being grown.

But even if we leave GMO seed aside, there are problems involved with eating corn. That's because corn creates huge blood sugar spikes. Corn is a major player, not just in promoting inflamed fat cells and accelerating FAT-flammation, but in damaging the intestinal tract as well. Think about it. Corn is used as feed for cattle and other animals, and why? Because it is a cheap feed. You may have heard that corn-raised beef creates a better steak? The reason is that corn makes a "fattier" cut of steak. **Corn is used to fatten up cattle and chickens. Why don't we realize that it is doing the same thing for humans?**

Corn is also high in omega-6, which helps create and perpetuate the imbalance in omega-3 and omega-6 fatty acids, a key factor in FATflammation. Remember, corn-fed beef is linked to heart disease, diabetes, cancer, as well as fat and obesity. Grass-fed beef is not. If you want to buy grass-fed beef, it will be advertised or promoted as pasteurized grass fed. Ask your butcher.

When I tell you that I think you should remove all products with corn from your diet, I'm not referring to a few pieces of freshly picked organic sweet corn that we all like to eat every summer. I'm talking about the hundreds of food products that contain highly inflammatory corn, most notably cornmeal, cornstarch, corn sweetener, corn oil, corn syrup, corn flour, and corn sugar. There are also corn-based food ingredients that don't include the word *corn*. I'm talking about ingredients like dextrose, dextrin, maltodextrin, vegetable gum, and xanthan gum. I highly recommend removing all products that include corn from your diet. To do this, you need to start reading food labels very, very carefully. As I've said several times already, probably the most difficult corn-derived ingredient to avoid is the potentially dangerous high-fructose corn syrup. If you want to get rid of your fat and you want to be healthy, HFCS and other corn products cannot be part of your life.

"Gluten Free" Does Not Mean Fatflammation Free

My friend Carolyn called me a couple of weeks ago, all excited because a gluten-free bakery had recently opened up in her town. "Isn't that great!?" she asked. I knew that Carolyn didn't have a real gluten sensitivity. She was interested in giving up gluten because she wanted to find an easy way to lose ten pounds. I didn't want to burst her bubble, but I also didn't want her to rush out and buy a loaf of gluten-free bread that would create even more FATflammation than your everyday whole wheat.

"Take a look at the labels," I suggested. "Find out what's in the products before you get too excited."

She called me back a few days later. "I'm so disappointed," she said. "One of the breads had white rice starch, potato starch, tapioca starch, xanthan gum, and a few other things. I think some sugar. I guess it's still fattening," she said.

"I'm afraid so," I told her. "And inflammatory."

In the last few years, many larger manufacturers have jumped on the "gluten free" bandwagon. So have many smaller bakeries. The food products they are marketing are free of gluten. It's good that manufacturers are taking the needs of people with celiac disease and true gluten sensitivity into account. I just wish they would try to manufacture foods that were healthy as well as gluten free. Also, like Carolyn, many of the people interested in buying these pastas and breads and cakes are not really sensitive to gluten. They are primarily interested in weight loss. Unfortunately, many of the products labeled "gluten free" are filled with ingredients that are inflammatory and create fat. These breads, cakes, cookies, muffins, and pastas usually contain corn, soy, white rice starch, potato starch, tapioca starch, sugar, and xanthan gum (there's more of that sneaky corn). These are not healthy choices

Because "gluten free" has become such a food manufacturer's buzzword, new replacements for wheat need to be found. Since corn is a cheap ingredient, guess what? Corn is often swapped for gluten in many gluten-free foods. I've even seen corn used in pasta.

SO THEN, CAN WE EAT ANY GRAINS?

Yes, of course. Grains can be included in a healthy diet, and there are many grains and cereals, as well as seeds that can be eaten in moderation. Notice the word *moderation*. The minute we start eating food made from grains or seeds of any kind, many of us can't stop. That's all we want to eat. We become fixated on our grains and forget about eating protein and vegetables. Some of us take our love of grains one step further. We remember to eat the protein and vegetables, but then also continue on to eat huge amounts of grains—which means that we are eating way too much food. Some of us love grains so much that it might be fair to say that we are addicted to them. This is a problem.

So what grains can we eat *in moderation*?

Brown Rice

Forget about white rice and focus on brown, a great and delicious grain. Unlike white rice, brown rice is not refined and includes all parts of the grain kernel—the bran, endosperm, and germ. Brown rice is also high in fiber, which will help you fight FATflammation, and it contains an abundant supply of several vitamins, minerals, and antioxidants. Numerous recent studies have shown that brown rice, a slow-release carbohydrate, can also help keep your blood sugar levels stable, another defense against FatFlammation. You can buy many different kinds of brown rice—long grain or short grain, for instance. Brown rice does take a little bit longer to cook than white rice but is well worth the extra effort. If you don't want to cook brown rice, you can also buy frozen brown rice, already cooked, in many natural food stores and supermarkets.

Oats

What's better than a bowl of oatmeal on a cold winter morning? The best and healthiest oats, are steel cut oats. Not only do they have the lowest glycemic index, steel cut oats are the least processed of all of the oat cereals. Steel cut oats are wonderful, but they do take about twenty to forty minutes to cook, depending on how chewy you want your oatmeal. If you absolutely don't have the time, choose old-fashioned rolled oats, which only take about ten minutes' cooking time. Oatmeal can also be made ahead of time and reheated. You can even take your oatmeal to work and reheat it. I absolutely do *NOT* recommend "instant oats," those little packets of oats that typically include sugar and salt. They are the most heavily processed, which automatically disqualifies them from a health and weight point of view. Don't even entertain the idea of adding these to your diet. This is inflammation in action.

Barley

Few people today take the time to cook a pot of barley, but every now and then, they should. Barley's biggest drawback is that it includes gluten. However, if you are not gluten intolerant, barley's advantages are numerous. High in vitamins B_1 (niacin) and B_3 (thiamine), barley is also high in selenium and magnesium, as well as other minerals and trace minerals. But barley's biggest health advantage is its incredibly high fiber content; in fact it has significantly more fiber than oats with fewer calories. Barley also helps keep your friendly gut bacteria even friendlier, which, as we know, is good for weight loss. Add barley to soups and stews, or cook it and then mix it with chopped veggies and a simple oil and lemon dressing to create a wonderful salad. Barley is easy to cook, though it does take longer than some of the other grains.

Quinoa

Everybody's favorite new whole grain is not really a grain or cereal. In fact, it's a seed, often referred to as a pseudocereal. Quinoa, which contains all the essential amino acids, is high in fiber and magnesium, as well as other important minerals. But best of all, quinoa is anti-inflammatory, which makes it one of your greatest allies in the fight against FATflammation.

Quinoa is easier to cook than rice. Combine it with vegetables and/or legumes, and a little bit of healthy oil for a fabulous meal. Or eat a bowl of quinoa on its own or as a cereal for breakfast. If you're not already eating quinoa as part of your regular diet, now is the time to start experimenting with all the ways to add quinoa into some of your meals.

Buckwheat

Buckwheat has been around for thousands and thousands of years. Delicious and gluten free, buckwheat is high in fiber and contains a variety of healthy phytonutrients, chemical compounds that occur naturally in plants and help combat all sorts of diseases—from inflammation and diabetes to strokes and even cancer. Buckwheat soba noodles are good in broth or as a side dish. They are also wonderful in cold summer salads with vegetables and a little bit of oil. Buckwheat flour makes good pancakes. Some of you may know buckwheat groats as kasha. If you decide to cook kasha, make sure you follow the directions, which may include coating the grains with egg whites. Otherwise, it all kind of mashes together. Kasha is a wonderful side dish that goes with many different foods.

Wild Rice

As you probably already know, wild rice is really a seed, as opposed to a true gain. It does not include gluten and has a reasonable amount of protein. It's also a good source of B vitamins, as well as other healthy minerals, including zinc. You can also combine wild rice with brown rice as a side dish. In fact, cooked wild rice combines well with a large number of vegetables to make delicious cold salads any time of year. I personally love wild rice. It has a delicious nutty taste and goes well with a variety of other foods.

Amaranth and Other Grains

Amaranth is typically referred to as a grain, but it's really a seed. Like quinoa, amaranth is closely related to spinach. With three times more fiber than wheat and more calcium than milk, amaranth is also a tremendous source of protein and is gluten free, which makes amaranth another fantastic ally in the fight against FATflammation. Amaranth flour can be used for breads, pitas, and pastas; amaranth can also be cooked as a hot cereal. It's also good toasted and sprouted and can be used to thicken sauces. One other surprising thing you can do with amaranth: it can be popped like popcorn, and who doesn't like that?

Millet and other grains such can also be part of a healthy diet. Such whole grains are great sources of the important and health-affirming B vitamins, phytonutrients, antioxidants, and fiber, all of which help fight against FATflammation.

Remember, though, to avoid at all costs every kind of refined grain—from wheat and corn to pasta and cereal—and enjoy whole grains regularly, but only in moderation.

PART THREE

THE FATFLAMMATION-FREE DIET PROGRAM

CHAPTER 9

STARTING A
FATFLAMMATION-FREE LIFE

*"I just want to be able to walk past a store window and not
want to cover my eyes. I want to feel good about how I look."*

*"I want to be able to walk up a couple of flights
of stairs without feeling as though I am huffing
and puffing. I want to be and feel healthy."*

*"I want to be able to fit in a ski jacket so I can go skiing again
without looking and feeling like a blimp coming down the hill."*

"I have young kids. I want to be able to keep up with them."

*"I want to be able to get up and dance
without feeling embarrassed."*

▶ Think about your own unique reasons for wanting to lose weight and get
rid of FATflammation. What is your personal "why"? Remind yourself of all
your own reasons. Yes, losing weight will help you feel healthier, more attrac-
tive, and more alive! But I would like you to go deeper than that and continue to ask yourself "WHY?" If your answer is "to get into that size 8 dress,"
or "so I never again have to shop in a 'stout' man's department and can throw
out all those shirts with X's on the size label" ask yourself, "Why do I want to
get into that size 8 dress?" or "Why do I want to throw out all those oversized shirts?" Keep asking until you know your core reasons for wanting to

lose weight. Then you will have your reasons on hand to remind yourself when motivation wanes or a strong food craving rears its ugly head. This will prevent you from slipping back into old patterns. Write your reasons down, and don't forget to remind yourself of your personal reasons on a regular basis. Doing this will help you achieve your goals.

Finally, no matter what your own personal goals are, I know that you don't want to feel as though your life is being controlled by your fat cells. The good news is that you can do this, and you can start doing it today!

MAKING THE COMMITMENT
AND TAKING CONTROL

Making smart decisions about food is one of the most reliable and easiest ways to take control of your life. The word *control* can sometimes have a negative connotation. However, right now, staying in control will help you create a direct path to success. You and I both know that the path to getting rid of FAT*flammation* isn't always going to be easy. However, planning ahead and being prepared is going to make it much easier. You wouldn't build a house without plans and blueprints. So read these sections carefully. Use them to help you create a solid and very achievable plan to help you reach your goal.

The FATflammation-Free Diet begins with an aggressive three-week program, designed to change the nature of your fat cells. Yes, you will have to stop eating the foods that create and fuel FATflammation, but you will have plenty to eat, and it won't be as difficult as you might think.

The men and women I've worked with are typically nervous about taking that first step and giving up some of the food they are accustomed to eating. They wonder whether they can sort of edge their way in. Here's a question I'm often asked: "Do I have to do everything at once? You know—add omega-3 and give up sugar. Can I do it a little bit at a time?" My answer is always the same. If you are sincere about wanting to get rid of FATflamamation, it's important to be very aggressive in the first few weeks.

Hesitation and skepticism are a natural part of trying anything new or taking a "leap" into unknown territory. It's been years, but I still remember when I decided to give up sugar for good. I realized what sugar was doing to my body and my health. So I made the jump into the unknown of a life without sugar or candy or cookies or cake. My first thoughts were, *How can I make it through the day without something sweet? Can I do this? Will I have enough energy if I'm not eating sugar?* I have to say that after the third day without sugar, what I saw happening seemed almost miraculous: my sugar cravings disappeared. Within a week I began to seriously lean-up; I looked and felt thinner; my energy level was through the roof; and I really felt good. To my shock and surprise, my cravings for all carbohydrates—not just sugar—began to disappear. This was all because I took that first cautious and doubtful, but nonetheless hopeful, step.

I see dramatic accomplishments every day with clients—men and women who have experienced profound changes in their weight and health. When they started out, most of them felt the pull of uncertainty. Yet they took that one step forward. One client I always remember, Karla, was a beautiful woman who weighed 305 pounds when she started working with me. She was miserable. Karla had joint pain, diabetes, back pain, and digestive issues. She couldn't sleep and was on medication for high cholesterol, insulin, and high blood pressure. Like so many, Karla was also genuinely addicted to sugar. But Karla made a strong decision to give up sugar and refined carbohydrates. She didn't wean herself; she did it cold turkey, all at once. Her results were amazing. By the end of the first week, she had already dropped five pounds; her joint pain diminished, her energy increased, and for the first time in years, she was able to sleep through the night. Karla was ultimately able to lose 170 pounds as well as get off her prescription medications! How is that for putting one foot into the cold water?

I've watched countless clients take the first step; I've seen them get healthy, shrink their fat cells, and lose weight. I knew they could do it, and I know you can do it. Taking that first step is critical because it says that you are taking action and that action means that you value yourself.

BEFORE YOU BEGIN:
KNOW YOUR FATFLAMMATION TRIGGERS

What triggers your eating sprees? All my clients have shared information about their triggers. Many of them told me that specific foods set them off; most shared emotional triggers that had them heading for their preferred overindulgence food. Some people associate food with certain activities; some regularly overindulge whenever they eat in specific places. Knowing what pushes your buttons helps you prepare for challenges, because when it comes to food, we all experience challenges.

Know Your Trigger Foods

We all have some special "trigger foods" that we have a difficult time resisting. These are the foods with which we form relationships best described as "addictive." Our triggers are typically fast food, fried foods, desserts, ice cream, chocolate, white bread, pasta, pizza, soda, and potato chips. They are sometimes junk foods or processed foods high in sugar, salt, and fat. Sometimes we form "addictive" relationships with foods that we may think of as healthy. Bananas, grapes, pineapple, raisins (high in sugar), peanut butter (high in salt), or corn chips are some examples. I personally have had to learn how to avoid crunchy little sticks made with ingredients such as seeds or oats and sold in natural food stores as "healthy snacks." If I didn't force myself to make a real effort, that "crunch" could be my downfall. The problem with the trigger foods we can't resist is that they can set off an avalanche of binge or addictive eating.

Food addiction is real. You may recall the comparison between sugar and cocaine. Both are addictive. Researchers found that when given the choice between sugar and cocaine, cocaine-addicted rats chose sugar. Both sugar and cocaine light up the same areas of the brain—the reward center. Also remember the gremlin ghrelin? High-sugar foods trigger ghrelin, a hormone that increases your appetite and stimulates cravings. Trigger foods are sometimes foods that you know are easily within your reach—such as that Chunky

Monkey in the freezer. You may think you can have just one bite, but you know from experience that taking even one bite might create a food frenzy. These are the foods that keep you stuck on the highway to Fatflammation. You have to let them go.

Know Your Trigger Places and Activities

While you are tossing out your trigger foods, get a better handle on your trigger places and activities. Do you, for example, have difficulty controlling your reactions to specific places like fast-food restaurants, donut shops, pizza parlors, or even coffee shops? Does something about the aroma or even ambience just draw you in and make you want to start ordering? Know this about yourself and stay away from these places. If your weakness (and addiction) is a sugar laden frappuccino, for example, don't agree to meet a friend for coffee at your favorite neighborhood coffee shop. Meet for a walk, meet in the park, or meet at the library. You just can't meet in a coffee shop until you've lost that addiction.

But maybe your favorite trigger places are located right in your own living room. Do you, for example, associate the couch with eating? Are you conditioned to chewing chips or popcorn while you watch television? If this is the case, know this about yourself so that you can recognize and resist your triggers. Change locations and start watching television while sitting in a chair, for example, or in your bedroom. I have actually convinced clients to get rid of specific items of furniture because they were so completely associated with eating. As you start changing your habits (or even your furniture), keep reminding yourself how important losing FATflammation is to your life. Don't hesitate to change small details in your environment in order to change your life for the better.

Know Your Trigger Emotions

Amy just had a phone argument with her best friend and she is still angry. She heads straight for the refrigerator, hesitating only a moment before opening the freezer door and taking out the container of her favorite ice cream, mint chocolate chip. *I shouldn't*

do this, she thinks, *but I'm so mad I don't care.* She opens the container, grabs a spoon, and, standing there in the kitchen, devours half a container. By the time she is finished eating, she is no longer angry at her best friend. She is angry at herself.

Carl is under stress. At work, too many projects require his attention, and he has dozens of deadlines. At home, he is concerned about his oldest son, who is having problems with math and he is worried about his wife, who is also working too hard. Many of us can identify with Carl's favorite method of handling stress: he grabs something to eat. On his way to work every morning, he stops and gets a couple of donuts and a large coffee into which he pours about six packets of sugar. He knows he shouldn't be doing it, but he feels as though he needs that "fix" to help him face the day. When he gets home, he has a large dinner, and then, even though he's not hungry, he looks for something else to eat. He likes things he can really get his teeth into—things that are hard, crunchy, and chewy, like some kind of chips or pretzels, which he washes down with soda or a beer. Carl knows that he is under stress, and he knows that he eats too much. But he doesn't really stop to connect his stress with his eating patterns.

Dina and her boyfriend broke up over a month ago, but she is still feeling very sad. In the days immediately following the breakup, she was so upset that she couldn't eat. That only lasted a few days. That's when she went on what she refers to as "my chocolate diet." At ten A.M. as she bites down on her third bar of Godiva chocolate for the day, she thinks, *I deserve this.* By noon, she is having a different set of emotions. She talks to herself, *My reactions are so predictable! Why am I being so self-destructive with the chocolate. It's bad enough "he" hurt me. Why am I hurting myself?*

The first time I spoke to Mallory about her eating habits, she acknowledged that her biggest food issue was "eating out of boredom." Whenever she didn't have anything to do, she would

immediately gravitate to the kitchen, where all her goodies were waiting. She wasn't hungry, she wasn't angry, she wasn't sad or depressed. She was just bored. Boredom was her primary emotion, and eating was her primary entertainment and diversion.

Do you eat more when you feel angry? Do you respond to an argument with somebody you love by heading straight to the refrigerator, like a homing pigeon? Emotions may trigger almost as much food intake (sometimes more) than hunger. For most of us, the term "comfort food" has serious meaning, and emotional eating can have serious consequences. Also, when you are eating to feed your stomach, you tend to stop when you full. When you are eating to feed your feelings, there is a tendency to just keep eating more and more. It is more difficult, after all, to satisfy your emotional needs than it is to satisfy your physical hunger.

A big problem with "feeding our feelings," as many of us know firsthand, comes from the guilt and self-blame experienced after we have indulged in emotional eating.

The first key to breaking these eating patterns is "awareness." Be very clear in your mind about what you are doing and why you are doing it. Each time you catch yourself looking for food because of an emotional trigger, remind yourself of your "why"—the primary reasons why you want to lose weight. If you still can't resist what you are feeling and absolutely must have something to eat, make sure that you always keep a bowl of cut-up veggies in your refrigerator for munching.

JOURNALING TO DOUBLE YOUR WEIGHT LOSS

Did you know that keeping a daily food diary or journal can actually double your weight loss? That's what one study that followed 1,700 participants for six months showed. Other studies have shown similar results. Keeping track of what you eat and how you feel about it helps you lose more weight.

Men and women with weight issues tend to indulge in "mindless" eating. Think about it. Are you busy and distracted much of the time? Are you sometimes so distracted that you fail to focus on what you eat, no matter how much you want to lose weight? If you are a contemporary "multitasker," you probably know what it is to grab bits of food here and there. Well, if you want to win your battle against FATflammation, your journal can be your best friend and biggest ally. Your journal will help you get a strong sense of what is helping or hindering you; you will be able to see, in black and white, what you eat every day. In this way, you become more aware of how you handle food—what you eat and why.

Journaling will also help you discover for yourself the benefits of being able to objectively analyze your relationship to food. Your issues with food represent an important area of your life, and a journal will help you realize the role food plays in your everyday life—from mindless eating to emotional eating. Journaling will also provide a constructive outlet for stress and anxiety, two often overlooked contributors to FATflammation. Many of my clients have told me that journaling reduces stress levels and makes them feel more in control and confident about how they are handling food.

Journaling helps you "know" and be aware of what you eat and drink; it will help you keep track of the supplements you take as well as document your food sensitivities, stress levels, exercise, and sleep. I ask all my clients to journal, and once they do, most of them never want to stop. Why? Because they see that it is making them more successful and confident!

Start by getting a journal that will fit into your briefcase, purse, or jacket pocket. You want to be able to take your journal with you everywhere you go so you have your "Accountability Assistant" with you at all times. The key to a successful journal revolves around being able to write things down immediately. Trying to later remember what you did or didn't eat or how you felt about it will not be effective.

The three primary requirements for journaling are honesty, commitment, and consistency. But it's also important to be kind to yourself. Don't beat yourself up over any self-perceived failing. At its heart, journaling is meant to help you learn more about yourself. View it as a gift.

On page one, list some of the reasons why you want to lost weight. What are your goals? Do you want to get healthier? Do you want to be able to wear clothes you love? Do you want to be able to go to that reunion and wear something that makes you look and feel good? Do you want to gain more confidence or have more energy to play with your children or grand-children? Do you simply want to feel better about yourself? It's good to write down *all* your reasons for wanting to lose weight. It's also good to read them regularly to remind yourself of what you want; this will help you remember to take yourself and your goals seriously.

Then write in your starting weight and your starting waist measurement, followed by your overall weight-loss goal. Once a week, weigh yourself and take your measurements. A word of caution, though: your weight will move up and down the scale for a number of different factors—from the amount of water you've drunk to the time of day or day of week you decided to step on the scale. Women also tend to retain water at different times of the month, and this can create ups and downs in weight. So fat loss is most effectively revealed in inches. After each weigh-in and measurement, write the results down in your journal. But make sure to do it on the same day of the week, and at the same time. If you start the FATflammation-Free Diet Program on a Sunday, for example, you will probably want to weigh yourself right before you begin, as soon as you wake up before you drink your water. Then, con-tinue to do your weekly weighing and measuring on Sunday morning.

Keeping Better Track of Your Body

Are you one of those people who keeps jumping on the scale to check exactly what's happening? Are you always nervously asking questions like, "Did I gain three ounces after lunch?" or "Did I weigh two ounces less before breakfast?" It's tempting to keep checking. I understand how you feel. But I want to tell you to stop doing that. Don't become a slave to your scale. Doing that isn't going to give you the information you want and it can confuse you and sabotage your efforts.

Measuring your waist is one of the best ways to assess true fat loss. Measuring your waist will also give you an idea about how much visceral or abdominal fat you have. Visceral fat is the dangerous fat that creates even more FATflammation. Abdominal fat increases your risk for cardiovascular disease, high blood pressure, "bad" cholesterol, insulin resistance, and diabetes. If you are male and your waist is forty inches or greater, you have a substantially greater risk of these health conditions. A woman with a waist circumference of thirty-five inches or more faces the same kind of risks.

So how do you measure yourself? It's very simple. All you need is an inexpensive soft fabric tape measure—the kind that is used to get measurements for sewing. Perhaps you already have one in a sewing kit. If not, you can find them online or in shops that sell sewing or knitting supplies. I found one in my local drugstore. Wrap it around your waist about one inch above your belly button. Take a look at the number and then write it down in your journal. That's it.

Another good journaling tip is to write down your list of trigger foods. Staying aware of what they are can help you avoid them. You might also want to write down your trigger emotions. Think about some of the situations that make you want to chow down. Do you eat more when you are sad, tired, or angry? Do you eat when you feel a sense of frustration? Do you eat when something goes wrong at work or when you argue with your significant other?

You can avoid eating at these times by recognizing these feelings when they occur.

Remember, too, to keep track of your meals. Write down everything you eat, including every snack or small piece of food you eat in between meals. Did you miss a meal or a snack? Write that down too. Jot down every beverage you drink throughout the day—and how much you drink.

Also take special note of your moods. Do you feel happy/stressed/ anxious/tired/energized? Regardless of how you feel, write it down.

Other things to note in your journal:

▶ Note whether you took your supplements or not.
▶ Note the type(s) of exercise such as cardio and strength training, including intensity of workout and how long you exercised.
▶ In the morning after you wake up, note how much and how well you slept.
▶ Did you plan each meal or snack in advance?
▶ Did you shop and do the prep so the appropriate foods were available to you?
▶ Do you have any items you need to add to your shopping list?
▶ How hungry were you before the meal or snack?
▶ How long did you wait between your meals?
▶ Did you pay close attention to portion sizes?
▶ Did you stop eating when you felt 80 percent full?
▶ Did you eat mindfully?
▶ Did you eat slowly?
▶ Did you avoid your trigger foods?
▶ Did you avoid sugar?
▶ Were you at home? Were you eating alone? Were you in a restaurant?
▶ Note your energy level.
▶ Did you practice mind-set techniques such as visualization?
▶ Note how your day was overall; was it great, successful, stressed, challenging?

Each night, before you go to bed, take the time to note all the ways in which you were successful for the day. Were you able to avoid refined carbohydrates? Congratulate yourself! This self-acknowledgment is very important in your overall success. So go ahead and pat yourself on the back. You deserve it! Also, if you experience any challenges during the day, add those as well.

DRINK YOUR WATER

If you are accustomed to eating and watching television, have some water on hand to drink while watching your favorite shows. Water is a powerful FAT-flammation fighter. Drinking water is also probably the very easiest strategy for reducing the size of your fat cells. It's so simple that it seems impossible that it could be so very true. But it is. Water can increase your metabolism and help you flush out the fat. We're talking water here. Not tea, soda, coffee, or juice. Just plain old-fashioned water. How easy is it to pick up a glass of water and swallow some down!? Start right now!

When we are even mildly dehydrated, we tend to lose our "thirst detectors." We don't recognize thirst for what it is and mistake what we are feeling for hunger. That's because the same area of the brain controls both hunger and thirst, and the signal it sends isn't specific enough to help you differentiate. We've all faced the dilemma of standing in front of the refrigerator feeling perplexed because we know we want something, but we're not sure what. We've also had the experience of eating too much food and still feeling hungry. Here's some advice: when this happens to you, drink a glass of water before you start putting food in your mouth. Most of the time, when you do this, your sense of wanting to eat—even though you're not really hungry—will go away. It usually takes about five minutes for this to happen.

Approximately 60 percent of your body is made up of water. It's the major component of most of your body parts. Even your brain and heart are more than 70 percent water. Every single cell, part, and process of your body needs water in order to stay alive and function. When cells aren't properly hydrated, cellular function slows down, and so does metabolism. This is why those who are even mildly dehydrated gain weight and feel tired. Also when you are dehydrated, your body responds by holding on to water. And what does that look like? Bloated belly, swollen ankles, fingers, and more. Conversely, when you drink more water, your body will start releasing the water it is holding, which makes water a natural diuretic.

And, no matter how mild, dehydration will automatically start the process of cellular inflammation. This means that every cellular process and function in your body, including your metabolism, will slow down. In particular, dehydration greatly impacts the function of your liver, which is your primary fat-burning organ, and your kidneys, as well as your entire digestive system. Drinking more water, for example, may help you deal with constipation. There also appears to be a correlation between mild dehydration and acid reflux, a condition that plagues so many people with FATflammation. Even mild dehydration can cause lethargy, fatigue, headaches, palpitations, foggy thinking, joint and muscle pain, as well as bloating. Some experts even go so far as to draw a direct correlation between chronic mild dehydration and chronic depression.

In addition, water keeps our electrolytes balanced, which is essential for cardiac health, and helps regulate testosterone levels—in both men and women. And, believe it or not, water can actually help you burn fat, because when you drink chilled or room-temperature water, your body promptly heats it up to body temperature, a thermogenic action that helps burn fat. Finally, because water helps flush out toxins, water can also help you win your battle against cellulite.

Remember, water helps you detox your body, which is an important key to reversing FATflammation. Water delivers more oxygen and nutrients to your cells; water helps your body get rid of toxins and waste. Drink your water so you will have happy, hydrated cells.

How much water should you be drinking each day? We are usually advised to drink half our body weight in ounces. That means that if you weigh 160 pounds, you should be drinking 80 ounces of water daily. That comes to about ten full glasses, spread out throughout the day.

Still, even if you feel completely lost without something to chew, be prepared with a bowl of fresh veggies. Think celery stalks, cauliflower florets, or endive. The important thing is that you prepare yourself for your impulses. You have developed habits that helped create FATflammation. Now you have to change them.

CHAPTER 10

STOCK YOUR KITCHEN WITH FATFLAMMATION-FREE FOOD

*"I hate looking around my kitchen and not being able
to find anything that I want to eat or that I'm allowed
to eat. When that happens, I always end up doing
something stupid like finding that old box of crackers in
the cupboard and eating them with strawberry jam."*

—BONNIE

▶ Most of us can identify with Bonnie. When you look in your refrigerator, pantry, or cupboard, it's essential that you be able to find FATflammation-free food. But before you go shopping, you first have to clean out your kitchen.

To prepare for the "new," we have to get rid of the old. Right this moment, you have food in your kitchen that will inevitably contribute to FATflammation. This food is sitting on the shelves of your refrigerator, freezer, pantry, and cupboards. You know it's gotta go. Nonetheless, you resist the idea of "tossing" it. I completely understand why you might feel that getting rid of "food" is wasteful and financially foolish. You may be asking yourself, *Do I really need to throw out that ketchup, even though it is made with high-fructose corn syrup? I don't use it that often . . . how bad can it be for me to have just a little of it every now and then?* I also understand why you may not want to throw out food you love. You may be thinking, *How will I feel if I don't have an emergency stash of frozen éclairs sitting in the back of the freezer?*

If you feel challenged by the act of tossing out "perfectly good food," you need to remember your ultimate goal. Stay laser focused on that. What you are doing is serious, and you need to take serious steps to get where you want to be.

Take a look at all the food labels in your kitchen. Remove any food that contains trans fats and/or partially hydrogenated oils (you can find these in a wide variety of foods, including margarine, frozen fried foods, baked goods—fresh and frozen—and candy. If you see the words, "partially hydrogenated," don't hesitate for a second. Just throw it out.

Remove all refined oils or oils high in omega-6 fats, foods loaded with corn, soy, peanut safflower, sunflower, and vegetable oil, a catchall term often used on soy oils.

Remove all foods that include any variety of sugar, including white sugar, brown sugar, date sugar, molasses, honey, agave syrup. While you're at it, get rid of any dried fruit such as raisins, dates, figs, and apricots.

Remove any products that have the words *high-fructose corn syrup* or *corn syrup* on the labels. You can find HFCS in jams, jellies, syrups, cookies, cakes, breads, muffins, mayonnaise, ketchup, tomato products, bottled drinks of all kind including sodas and juice drinks. They have to go. This is a nonnegotiable.

Remove all artificial sweeteners and anything that includes artificial sweeteners.

Remove all white rice, pasta, crackers, cookies, cakes, white bread, English muffins, as well as anything that includes any refined carbohydrates such as white flour or tapioca starch.

Remove anything that includes corn or cornmeal. Check breads, muffins, cake mixes, and so on.

Remove all soy products that are not fermented. Read your labels. Soy is in many foods including some breads, muffins, butter substitutes and, of course, tofu and soymilk.

Remove all processed foods.

Finally, don't cheat: Make sure you have removed all your personal "trigger" foods.

The kitchen is not the only place we keep food. Do you have sweet snacks tucked away in your car, your desk at work? How about your bedside table? It's absolutely essential to keep foods you know you can't resist out of all parts of your life, including your fridge, your desk, your pantry, your purse, and your closet.

Getting the food you don't want to be eating out of your life is a big step, but you have to do what you have to do to beating FATflammation. It sometimes helps if you get a friend or relative to help you clean out your kitchen and your life.

Once you're free of the bad foods, you can stock up on the good food. Start by reading over the diet plans and menus for all three weeks. Read these sections over at least twice. Become comfortable with the kind of foods that you will be eating. This is important. When you have read all these sections twice, go back and focus on the food and menus for Week One.

People have different opinions about grocery shopping. You either love it or hate it. Personally I love it because I find it relaxing. It also makes me feel as though I am doing something proactive for my health. Nonetheless, I always take a shopping list. Going to the store without a list of foods that will help you reverse FATflammation is like taking a sailboat out to sea without a rudder. Venturing out unprepared, you are at the mercy of the waves, the wind, and the environment. Without a list, you are at the mercy of the way food is marketed and presented. The list will keep you from being pulled hither and yon by TODAY'S SPECIALS and VISIT OUR BAKERY signage along with beautiful displays. You probably know what it's like going to the supermarket when you're hungry and not really sure what you want to buy. Everything looks scrumptious and delectable and so it goes into the basket. Then you arrive home and discover that you have bought quite a few things you shouldn't be eating.

It's easy to fall victim to packaging and displays and fill our carts with things we really don't intend to buy. We see that package of chocolate chip cookies, and we think, *Oh I'll only eat one.* Or *It will be good to have something in the house in case somebody stops by,* or *My husband, daughter, son, mother, father, sister, brother, cousin, friend would like that.* Something I always tell my clients; *IF YOU*

BRING IT HOME FROM THE GROCERY STORE, ASSUME IT WILL GO IN YOUR MOUTH.

A shopping list will help you stay centered; it will help you stay in control; it will help you resist buying food you shouldn't be eating.

CHOOSING HEALTHY OILS

Your battle against FATflammation begins with your decision to choose only healthy anti-inflammatory oils and fats. One of the first things I do with every new client is give them a thorough "oil check." How much do you know about the oils you have been eating? For example, do you usually keep prepared salad dressings in the refrigerator? What are the ingredients? When you take out container of food from the nearest grocery store or delicatessen, do you ask what kind of oil is being used? Do you have any idea what kind of oils your favorite restaurants use? Do you ask your server?

Here are some things to remember when shopping.

Olive Oil

Everyone needs to keep a good bottle of extra-virgin olive oil (EVOO) in their kitchen. Not only does it fight FAT*flammation,* it also reduces our chances of developing heart disease. Olive oil is an excellent monounsaturated fat, which means that it is high in healthy monounsaturated fatty acids (MUFA). It's particularly high in oleic acid—a good fat that raises your HDL (good cholesterol) and lowers LDL (bad cholesterol). It's also a source of polyphenols and antioxidants, including vitamin E.

When choosing olive oil, read the labels carefully. Here's some help in understanding what the labels mean:

Extra-virgin olive oil is the highest grade of olive oil. It comes from the first pressing and includes no refined oil. The acidity level is no more than 0.8%. This is the preferred olive oil.
Virgin olive oil is the next grade of olive oil. Its acidity level is no more than 2%. This is okay, but not ideal.

> **Pure Olive oil is a blend and includes some refined oil as well as virgin or extra-virgin olive oil. I don't recommend it.**
>
> **Olive Oil is a blend of virgin oil and refined oil. I don't recommend it.**
>
> **Light Olive Oil is a refined olive oil. It does not mean that the oil has fewer calories or a lower fat, but it does have less taste. I don't recommend it.**

Important: Olive oil should always be purchased in a dark, opaque bottle. Exposure to light can oxidize the oil causing it to turn rancid. Olive oil is best when it hasn't been touched by heat. When cooking with any oil, it should not be heated beyond its smoke point. With olive oil, you reach that temperature somewhere between 375 and 400 degrees.

Only Use Fresh Oils

If an oil, even a "good" oil, has started to turn rancid, it can exacerbate FAT-flammation. Usually rancid oil starts to smell a little strange. Most oils have "sell by" or "use by" dates. Once a bottle of olive oil is opened, for example, make sure that it is stored in a dark container out of the light. I use olive oil frequently so I rarely keep it that long. But to avoid rancidity, if it smells "funny" or if it has been open for more than a few months, it's probably wisest to toss it.

What happens when oil goes rancid? You've seen an apple turn brown? This is oxidation in action and that same process happens to oil. Oils that are exposed to too much heat, light, or oxygen will create a storm of rancid or oxidized fat. Eating rancid oil damages your cells and contributes to FAT*flammation*.

Coconut Oil

For years, many of us avoided coconut oil because we were told that it was a saturated fat that contributed to heart disease. We now know that coconut oil seems to improve cardiac health and increases the amount of HDL (good cholesterol) in our blood. Coconut oil contains medium chain fatty acids (MCFAs), which are delivered to the liver where they are converted to energy as opposed to being stored as fat. Coconut oil also improves thyroid function, and boosts sluggish metabolism. One study showed that women who ate approximately two tablespoons of coconut oil every day had less belly fat at the end of a 12-week period.

Coconut oil is also rich in lauric acid, which will boost your immune system as well as your metabolism. This is absolutely one of my go-to oils.

When you go looking for coconut oil on your grocery store shelves, you will probably find it in the section devoted to health foods. You may also find a product called Coconut Butter which is slightly different.

Coconut oil—The oil that is extracted from coconuts.
Coconut butter—The meat of the coconut.

Coconut oil is good for cooking because it can handle higher heat without smoking. When an oil starts to smoke during cooking, this sends a signal that the structure of the fat is changing and becoming inflammatory. You can use it, for example, in baked goods or as a substitute for butter or olive oil on vegetables. Both coconut oil and coconut butter are great on baked sweet potato.

Both coconut oil and coconut butter are solid at room temperature and actually look like shortening when cold. In the winter months, you may need to scoop out the amount you need. It melts quickly if you want to use it for cooking. In the summer coconut oil tends to liquefy; don't be surprised if it looks like a jar of water. Solid or melted, coconut oil is a highly effective and healthy fat-burning oil.

When buying this oil, choose organic expeller pressed and extra virgin.

Macadamia Nut Oil

This tree nut oil is the new kid on the block in terms of its health benefits. I now think of it as one of my very favorite oils. It's very high in oleic acid, which helps reduce FATflammation and is even higher in beneficial monounsaturated fats than olive oil. It has a high smoke point—close to 410 degrees, which means that you can use it for most cooking without it degrading. It also tastes good on salads; I use it on salads almost every day.

Butter

Yes, butter. Many of us remember being told to "give up" butter for heart health, but recent studies have shown little association between saturated fat and heart disease. Butter also contains high concentrations of butyrate and helps promote a healthy gut. One of the greatest things about butter is that it tends to make us feel satiated when we eat it. Ideally, you should be buying butter from cows that are grass fed. Grass-fed butter is anti-inflammatory and provides a nutritional boost for your body. So how do you find grass-fed butter? There are several choices:

Are there any nearby local dairies that produce milk from grass-fed cows? Check local listings and also check your local farmers' markets. Even if nobody sells it, some of the farmers may know how to find it. Visit a store that specializes in natural food, such as Whole Foods and see what is available. Some dairies that produce organic milk also sell butter from cows that graze in pastures. Organic Valley is one example. Some butters imported from Ireland, such as Kerry Gold, are produced from cows that are out grazing for most of the year. Many grocery stores now carry this. New Zealand also exports some fine butters which are grass fed and organic.

What you don't want to buy is butter from cows that are getting GMO grains, hormones or antibiotics. Not all organic dairies leave their cows out to pasture, but organic brands guarantee that at least the cows are getting feed that is pesticide and GMO free.

OILS YOU ABSOLUTELY DON'T WANT TO BUY OR USE

There are several reasons why I don't want you to buy or eat certain oils or salad dressings or other food products that include the following oils. Primarily, of course, I want you to get rid of FATflammation. This means that you have to eat fewer fats that are high in Omega-6 because these foods disrupt the Omega-3/Omega-6 balance and help create FATflammation. I also want to you to avoid foods that use genetically modified products, and I also want you to stay away from foods that have been processed in such a way that they include unhealthy additives and chemicals.

Here's a List of Oils I Don't Want You to Use

Canola oil

Corn oil

Vegetable oil

Palm oil or Palm kernel oil

Peanut oil

Soybean oil

Sunflower oil

Safflower oil

Grapeseed oil

Margarine

Any fake butter or vegetable oil products such as "I Can't Believe It's Not Butter" or Smart Balance.

Trans fats

Anything that has "partially hydrogenated" listed on the ingredient list

Any commercial salad dressing that has one of these oils listed on the ingredient list, particularly when they it is high up on the list.

I realize how challenging it can be to find foods that don't include some of these oils. But it can be done. Read labels carefully. If an omega-6 oil is at the top of the list, let it go.

A note: I realize how challenging it can be to find foods that don't include some of these oils. But it can be done. Read labels carefully. If an Omega-6 oil is at the top of the ingredient list, let it go.

A Special Note About Canola Oil

If you do an internet search about canola oil, you will find dozens of opinions about its health benefits or lack thereof. Some people will tell you that an ingredient in canola oil also has industrial uses, such as insect repellant. You may also hear that the manufacture of canola oil involves chemicals that are less than desirable for food use. Others will assure you that canola oil is high in oleic acid, which is very good for the health of your heart. It is all quite confusing.

Personally I'm not a fan of canola oil. Why? Because it's a genetically engineered product created from the toxic rapeseed plant. It's highly refined, going through a multi-step process of bleaching and refining at high temperatures. Because it tends to have a strange odor, it also requires a process of deodorization to make it taste and smell fresh. The bottom line: I don't think canola oil, which is now found in just about everything, has been around long enough for us to be certain that it is healthy and beneficial. Some experts also believe that canola oil falls into the category of a trans fat. I don't use it and don't recommend using it.

Trans Fats—The Very Worst Oils

Trans fats are created by a process called hydrogenation—where they turn liquid oil into solid fat. Today, even some fast food restaurants have banned the use of trans fats in any of their fried foods sold in the U.S. Trans fats, also called "partially hydrogenated oils" are terrible for us, and just about everyone now acknowledges it. I have been warning people about the dangers of trans fats for years and am happy that the food industry is finally acknowledging the seriousness of the problem. Unfortunately, just about everybody has had an encounter or two with trans fats. Who hasn't eaten a Twinkie or two, not to mention movie popcorn or fast food French fries? Nonetheless, it's never too late to change your eating patterns and reverse any poor choices from your past.

The history of transfatty acids illustrates how our health can be damaged when the food industry decides to emphasize and promote man-made alternatives to old-fashioned whole foods as provided by nature. It's important to remember that trans fats were once considered a good thing—a reasonable alternative to butter. The first widespread use of trans fats took place during World War II when consumers began using trans-fat-laden margarine as an alternative to the more expensive butter. Food manufacturers quickly discovered that not only were trans fats a less expensive ingredient, they also extended food product shelf life. Trans fats are comparable to plastic bags in that they don't spoil or degrade for a very long time. When you are tempted to eat something that includes trans fats, ask yourself. Do I want to be eating something that resembles plastic instead of real food?

In the 1990s, medical experts began to realize that trans fats were creating huge health-related problems, including obesity and heart disease. As far as fats are concerned, these highly toxic fats are the worst of the worst. They help FAT*flammation* flourish, slow down metabolism, clog arteries, and are considered a major contributor to heart disease. If you want your bad cholesterol numbers to go up, and your good cholesterol number to go down, just go out and indulge in foods that contain these lethal fats. They are so bad for our health that, since 2006, food manufacturers in the U.S. have been required to warn consumers by listing trans fats on all ingredient labels. Also in 2006, New York City became the first city in the nation to ban trans fats in all restaurant foods. As a matter of fact (and fat), they have been proven to be so bad for you that the FDA is moving closer to banning *all* trans fats from *all* foods sold in the U.S. In the meantime, trans fats are still found in a variety of foods.

If you read your labels, you will also notice that the labels on many foods today specifically say "No Trans Fats." Consumers need to realize that this sentence can be deceptive. Food manufacturers are allowed to say "0 Trans Fats" so long as the food includes less than 0.5 grams of trans fats per serving. But if you are eating more than one serving—say three cookies instead of the two listed as a serving size, those trans fats will be adding up. Read your ingredient labels carefully. If there are trans fats in the food, you will see them listed as "partially hydrogenated" oils. If you are eating in a restaurant, take the time to ask if they are using trans fats in their cooking oils. If they are, order something that does not include any of these dangerous oils or go someplace else.

The verdict is in: STAY AWAY FROM TRANS FATS!

The Fatflammation-Free 3-Week Shopping List

Here are some of the things that belong on your list. (See the FATflammation-Free Complete Foods List in the appendix for other options.)

OILS

Cold-pressed extra-virgin olive oil
Macadamia nut oil
Coconut oil (organic, virgin, unrefined)

CANNED FISH

Water-packed wild salmon   *Sardines*
Water-packed light tuna   *Anchovies*
Water-packed tuna packets

JUICES

Low-sodium vegetable juice (preferably organic)
Low-sodium tomato juice

LEGUMES

Lentils   *Kidney beans*
Garbanzo beans   *Cannellini beans*
Black beans

SOUPS AND SAUCES

Low-sodium marinara sauce (Read the ingredients and avoid those with
 sugar or HFCS.)
Canned low-sodium lentil soup
Low-sodium chicken broth
Chopped tomatoes

GRAINS

Steel-cut oatmeal

Brown rice (if you don't want to cook your own, you can find frozen cooked brown rice in many supermarkets and natural food stores)

Wild rice

Quinoa

Brown rice penne pasta

NUTS, SEEDS, AND NUT BUTTERS

Almonds

Walnuts

Pistachios

Cashews

Chia seeds

Almond butter

CONDIMENTS AND SPICES

Cinnamon powder

Taco seasoning (Look for MSG and additive-free mixes or make your own; there are many recipes online.)

Chili powder

Oregano

Cumin

Salsa

Pico de gallo

Balsamic vinegar

Red wine vinegar

Sun-dried tomatoes

Olives

Apple cider vinegar

FROZEN FOODS

Frozen berries

Frozen spinach (an alternative to fresh spinach)

PERISHABLES

Take another look at the menus and recipes to see what you will preparing and eating.

DAIRY

Yogurt

You will be eating ½ cup of yogurt each day. Choose between plain, unsweetened 2 percent regular or Greek yogurt or plain coconut yogurt. If you buy a 32-ounce container of yogurt, you should have enough for eight days. If you want to use coconut yogurt one day and regular yogurt the next, that's fine. You will be having yogurt every day for three weeks. Check the expiration dates.

Butter (preferably from grass-fed pastured cows)
Almond milk
Coconut milk
Cheese (Weeks Two and Three; check menus)

EGGS

You will need almost a dozen eggs each week. Most egg-laying chickens, even free range, are fed some grains so if possible, buy eggs that are labeled pasture raised and organic, which means they will not have been fed superinflammatory GMO feed. Don't forget to check out your local farmers' markets for eggs that are pasture raised.

MEAT

Boneless, skinless chicken breast
Chicken breast (bone in)
Ground turkey
Turkey thighs
Turkey bacon
Turkey sausage
Grass-fed steak (4–6 ounces)
Grass-fed ground beef
(or ground buffalo)

If you want to limit your shopping trips for meat, any of these meat choices can be purchased ahead of time, frozen, then defrosted as needed.

SLICED MEATS

Roast beef

Turkey

Chicken

Prosciutto (nitrate free)

FRESH SEAFOOD

Cod

Tuna (fresh)

Salmon

Shrimp

Scallops

FRESH VEGETABLES

Avocados

Mushrooms

Tomatoes

Asparagus

Spinach

Salad greens—all varieties
   (arugula, romaine,
   watercress, mixed greens)

Bell peppers

Onions

Garlic

Kale

Zucchini

Celery

Cauliflower

Broccoli

Cucumber

Green beans

Sweet potatoes

Spaghetti squash

Parsley

FRESH FRUIT (Fruit has a limited shelf life, so shop accordingly.)

Fresh lemons (Take another look
   at the weekly plans. You will
   use a lot of lemons, so don't
   skimp.)

Fresh berries (These don't keep
   well, so either use frozen or only
   buy enough for a few days.)

Kiwis (Check your menu plan to
   see what days you will be eating
   kiwis, and shop accordingly.)

Apples

Pears

Grapefruit

Peaches

DIPS (Buy prepared or see later recipes to make your own.)

Guacamole   Lentil

Hummus   Black bean

WRAPS AND ALLOWED BREADS

Coconut wraps   Whole-grain pita pockets

Brown rice wraps   Brown rice pita pockets

Low-carb, high-fiber tortillas   Gluten-free sprouted English muffins

MISCELLANEOUS

Fresh or jarred pesto   Teas (such as green tea, Rooibos,

Chai tea bags   Pu-Erh)

TRACKING YOUR FOOD SENSITIVITIES

Because food sensitivity or intolerance can be a contributing factor in FAT-flammation, I'd like for you to be aware of any foods to which you might be sensitive. A food intolerance or sensitivity generally shows itself via a reaction caused by antibodies known as immunoglobulin G (IgG). Symptoms typically appear anywhere from several hours to three days after eating the offending food. If you are sensitive to a specific food or food group, the most common reactions include digestive disturbances such as bloating, diarrhea, or gas. Some people also get headaches or a sense of being congested. Other common reactions include muscle aches, insomnia, fatigue, low energy, rashes, acne, or other skin conditions. If you have serious food allergies or sensitivities, you probably already know what they are. Some of the most common food sensitivities include: corn, dairy, soy, and gluten.

The FATflammation-Free Diet Program cuts out all corn and soy during all three weeks. If you are sensitive to any of these foods, you will begin to feel better within days.

On Week One, you will be giving up all gluten as well as other grains.

On Week One, you will also be giving up all dairy except yogurt, because most people who are sensitive to dairy are typically still able to eat yogurt. However, if you think or know that you are sensitive to dairy, you can choose coconut yogurt, which also contains beneficial cultures.

If you are sensitive to gluten, dairy, or other grains, you should start feeling better within a few days.

By the end of Week One, you will have gone seven days without corn, soy, gluten, and dairy, except for yogurt. If you have food sensitivities, many, if not all, of your symptoms should have lessened or disappeared. Now it's time for you to figure out which are the offending foods.

On Week Two, you will add some regular dairy, such as cheese, back into your diet. When you start eating dairy again, if you notice that you are having symptoms associated with food sensitivity, they will typically appear within three days of eating a dairy product. If you believe you are experiencing problems eating dairy, stop eating dairy and substitute another protein.

On Week Three, several foods that include gluten will be reintroduced into your diet. If you experience symptoms, this tells you that "gluten has gotta go" permanently from your life.

I realize some people are sensitive to eggs. Nonetheless, I have included eggs because adults have usually outgrown their sensitivity to eggs. Also, people who have problems eating eggs usually already know about it. If you think or know that eating eggs triggers any kind of reaction or discomfort, do not eat them. Instead, swap them out for any other good *protein* source. Think about eating poultry or fish. You need protein so *don't* substitute cereal or carbohydrates. People who have problems eating eggs should become accustomed to eating foods for breakfast that are more commonly associated with lunch or dinner. Smoothies that include other sources of protein such as whey or pea-rice protein are also good choices.

CHAPTER 11

THE FATFLAMMATION-FREE DIET
3-WEEK PROGRAM

*"It's time for you to jump-start your fat loss by giving up all
those toxic foods that have given you inflamed fat cells. It's time
for you to eat only 'clean' foods that will reduce inflammation
and balance your omega-3/omega-6 fatty acids. So say
good-bye to all those inflamed fat cells and get moving on the
FATflammation-Free Highway toward your ideal weight."*
—DR. LORI

▶ Before you begin, make certain that you are prepared. Read over the
daily menus presented later in the book very carefully. Read the recipes and
diet suggestions. Be absolutely certain that you understand the basic elements of a FATflammation-Free Meal. Have you removed all the food that
you shouldn't be eating from your environment? Did you do your shopping?
Do you have food you should be eating available and ready?

A Word about Prepping and Planning

Planning for the week ahead is going to make it much, much, much easier to reach your goals. I have had clients who succeeded in losing the
twenty pounds they wanted to lose, and I have had clients who succeeded in losing the one hundred to two hundred pounds they wanted

to lose. The one quality all these successful clients shared is that they made the commitment to planning their meals ahead, and they did the necessary preparation. You know how it is with food. If you don't have what you should be eating handy and available, you tend to grab something you shouldn't be eating.

Make "Prepping for the Week" your motto. It takes just a bit of time to make enough hard-boiled eggs for the week, for example. It doesn't take that long to wash and prepare enough salad greens for several days. Don't hesitate to cook and freeze some meals ahead. If you work, snack and lunch time can be a FATflammation disaster. I suggest that you plan to take your lunch to work. If you don't have one already, buy a small insulated bag or cooler and some cold packs to keep in the freezer. Preparing your lunch meals at home the night before will make it all doable. Don't allow yourself to be without prepared food at work, confronting the temptations of a vending machine and the coffee wagon. However, that being said, if you do get caught without your lunch, part of planning and preparing is to stock in your desk nonperishable snacks and foods such as canned wild salmon, nuts, and seeds as your emergency stash that you can eat in a pinch.

Planning and preparing includes some cooking. Cooking gives you ultimate control over what goes into your mouth. Just always make sure that you have the food you need ready to be prepared.

And don't ever be without your bottle of water!

YOUR TYPICAL FATFLAMMATION-FREE DAY— ALL THREE WEEKS

Drink a cup of lemon water (juice of ½ lemon in hot/warm water) as soon as you wake up

Drink two (8-ounce) glasses of water before breakfast

Breakfast

Take your supplements

Midmorning snack

Drink two (8-ounce) glasses of water before lunch

Lunch

Midafternoon snack

Drink two (8-ounce) glasses of water with 1 teaspoon cider vinegar before dinner

Dinner

WHAT WILL YOU WILL BE EATING?

Starting a new diet raises many questions. I know that almost all my clients ask me two specific questions: "What can't I eat?" and "What can I eat?" Here is a general overview of the foods excluded and included in the FATflammation-Free Diet Program.

FOOD THAT YOU WILL NOT BE EATING IN ANY OF THE THREE WEEKS

Corn

Soy

Sugar (all forms)

Inflammatory omega-6 oils—corn, soy, peanut, safflower, sunflower, and "vegetable." (Vegetable oil is a catchall term often used on soy oils.)

Canola oil

Trans fats (any food product that includes the words "partially hydrogenated" on the label)

Refined grains (white bread, pasta, white rice)

Artificial sweeteners

Any foods that include HFCS

Some high-starch vegetables such as white potatoes

FOOD THAT YOU WILL BE EATING

Protein

You will give your sluggish metabolism an immediate boost by including a good source of protein with every meal and snack.

Animal protein choices

Lean meats such as chicken, turkey, beef, or lamb are allowed in all three weeks. Whenever possible, you should be choosing grass-fed meat and free-range poultry.

Free-range organic eggs. Unless you have a food sensitivity to eggs, these are allowed in all three weeks. If possible, buy eggs from free-range chickens. Organic is always preferable because it guarantees that the hens were not fed GMO grains.

Most varieties of fish and seafood, including salmon, shrimp, cod, flounder, sardines, tuna, anchovies, sole, scallops. You can choose fresh or canned and packed in water. Don't buy farm-raised fish unless you know it is from a trusted supplier.

Dairy

The only dairy products allowed during Week One are yogurt and whey protein. If you determine that you are not sensitive to dairy, other dairy products such as cheese will be added back into your diet for Weeks Two and Three.

Fats

Healthy fat burns fat! So you will be adding healthy fats such as coconut oil, olive oil, and macadamia nut oil to every meal. You will also be eating fatty fish, nuts, and or seeds. Don't be afraid of healthy fat. You will also be eating some beef, and, once again, I encourage you to use grass-fed beef whenever possible.

Grains

Week One: You will not be eating any grains.

Week Two: You will continue to avoid those grains that contain gluten such as whole wheat. However, you will be eating brown rice, quinoa, wild rice, and oatmeal.

Week Three: If you are not gluten sensitive, you will be adding some whole wheat products into your diet along with the brown rice, quinoa, wild rice, and oatmeal.

Other Carbohydrates

Vegetables

You are allowed unlimited amounts of nonstarchy veggies such as spinach, asparagus, kale, peppers, mushrooms, all varieties of lettuce, celery, cucumber, and so on.

You are allowed *limited* amounts of high-starch, high-fiber vegetables such as sweet potatoes, yams, and squash.

Fruits

You are allowed two portions a day of low-sugar/high-fiber fruits such as most berries, kiwi, apple (preferably Granny Smith), grapefruit, and peaches.

WHAT WILL YOU BE DRINKING?

Water

Drink a minimum of half your body weight in ounces each day. This includes the two full glasses of water before each meal. (If you weigh 160 pounds, half of that comes to 80 ounces. 80 ounces of water = 10 [8-ounce] glasses.) Remember that drinking two glasses of cool/cold water before each meal will automatically boost your metabolism.

Lemon Water

One of the recommendations that I make for weight-loss success is to have a cup of soothing lemon water first thing in the morning. The water can be cool, warm, or hot. It will immediately boost your metabolism and help detox your liver (your number one fat-burning organ). Lemon helps the liver break down fat; lemon contains lots of vitamin C to help quash liver inflammation and oxidation; and lemon water can help reduce bloating and prevent cravings. Lemon also contains pectin. A 2007 study showed that beverages containing pectin helped keep the participants in the study feel fuller, longer. Squeeze half a lemon into a mug of warm/hot, or even cool water. If you like the taste of lemon, add more.

Water with apple cider vinegar

Like lemon juice, raw organic apple cider vinegar helps balance blood sugar levels. Once again, remember that balanced blood sugar means fewer cravings and hunger pangs. Organic apple cider vinegar (such as Bragg's) is a fermented product. Fermented foods and probiotics are important tools in the battle against FATflammation. Apple cider vinegar also contains pectin. A study done in 2009 showed that those who consumed vinegar had substantially greater overall weight loss—as well as greater loss of abdominal fat—than the placebo group. Just add 1 teaspoon to 1 tablespoon of organic apple cider vinegar to the water you are drinking before dinner.

Optional fluids

You are allowed coffee, black tea, green tea, herbal teas such as Rooibos, and stevia-sweetened sodas.

Sweeteners

Some people cannot do without adding some sweeteners to beverages such as coffee and tea. Some allowed sweeteners are (for a more complete list, see page 228):

Stevia

Xylitol (When buying Xylitol, be sure to buy only noncorn, non-GMO Xylitol. Look for Xylitol made from white birch.)

Yacon syrup (Yacon syrup, which tastes a little like molasses, is also a

prebiotic and good for your digestive tract.) A study done in 2009 showed that daily consumption of yacon syrup contributed to a decrease in weight as well as waist circumference.

The Power of Tea

Several teas can help boost your fat loss. Here are some of them:

Green Tea

All tea is healthy, but green tea seems to run ahead of the pack in terms of its healthful and weight-loss benefits. Green tea contains the antioxidant epigallocatechin gallate (EGCG); numerous studies show its benefit in fighting fat. It helps shrink your fat cells and you! It is also helpful in treating and preventing various diseases. Green tea contains the amino acid L-theanine that exerts an antistress effect while increasing dopamine—a "feel-good" neurotransmitter.

Green tea boosts your metabolism, fat oxidation, and energy levels. It balances blood sugar and helps stop cravings. Add lemon juice to further enhance its fat-burning effects. Green tea contains caffeine but not as much as coffee.

Pu-Erh Tea

A mild Chinese tea, pu-erh (pronounced "pu-air") is actually fermented. Therefore it's high in beneficial bacteria (probiotics) that help reduce gut inflammation and therefore weight loss. This makes it another perfect tea accompaniment to the FATflammation-Free Diet Program. Used mainly for weight loss, it boosts metabolism and promotes lower cholesterol. It contains caffeine.

Rooibos

Rooibos (pronounced "roy-ee-boss"), a South African herb, is not only rich in inflammation-fighting antioxidants, it also helps to promote a healthy fat-burning liver and helps prevent the much too prevalent fatty liver associated with poor diets and weight gain. Rooibos helps keep the pesky fat-creating hormone cortisol low and helps promote a healthy digestive tract. It contains no caffeine.

SUPPLEMENTS THAT FIGHT FATFLAMMATION

Many Americans are deficient in important nutrients and need additional vitamins. The lack of nutrients contributes to inflammation, weight gain, poor immunity, insulin resistance, low energy levels, and mood and digestive problems. There are also several supplements that help fight FATflammation. Take a good look at the complete supplement list on page 212. Ideally I would like you to take all the recommended supplements. However, I do understand that you might be reluctant to rush out and buy everything on the list.

If your budget only allows a certain number of supplements, choose the six recommended below. If you can purchase only one supplement, make it omega-3 fish oil for reversing inflamed fat cells and thus reversing FATflammation. IMPORTANT: Take all your supplements except the glucomannan fiber after you have eaten to prevent digestive distress. It's also important to note that when you take supplements without food, they are not effective and it's a waste of money. I suggest taking glucomannan, which is a fiber, not a supplement, thirty minutes before meals. It can be included in one of your 8-ounce glasses of water.

Omega-3 fish oil	4,000 milligrams daily
Multivitamin + mineral (choose one without iron)	
Probiotic (multistrained)	one capsule, 15 billion CFUs (colony-forming units) daily
Vitamin D3	3,000 to 4,000 IUs daily
Chromium picolinate*	400 micrograms daily
Glucomannan fiber*	2.5 grams to 5 grams 30 minutes before a meal
*Important help for fighting hunger and cravings	

Many people who go on the FATflammation-Free Diet Program report that most, if not all, of their cravings for refined carbohydrates such as sugar, bread, and pasta begin to disappear within a few days. However, if you worry about feeling hungry or having cravings, I especially recommend that you try chromium picolinate and glucomannan fiber.

Chromium Picolinate

This mineral often helps stop sugar and carbohydrate cravings. Studies indicate that chromium picolinate can decrease body fat and increase lean muscle mass while balancing blood sugar

Glucomannan

Glucomannan is a fiber supplement that is highly effective in promoting a sense of fullness while helping to control food cravings. The brand I take is PGX, but many others are available. Be sure to follow the product instructions. My clients typically feel that this additional fiber has been extraordinarily helpful in terms of losing weight. **IMPORTANT!** Make absolutely sure that you drink the recommended water requirement in order to prevent constipation.

An Important Word about Fiber

Studies show that if you include more fiber in your diet, you're going to be leaner and less likely to get overfat. Adding fiber will also help you feel as though you've had more than enough to eat. This means that you are more likely to lose weight. Fiber also helps slow the rate at which food enters your bloodstream, which translates into balanced blood sugar levels. Another good thing: when your blood sugar is balanced, cravings typically start disappearing. It also takes longer to feel hungry again after a meal that is higher in fiber. Fiber does something else that helps in your fight against FATflammation. Like a superefficient broom, it works its way through your digestive system, sweeping toxins out of your gut.

There are two types of fiber—soluble and insoluble. Both are important. Soluble fiber is easily dissolved in water. Sources of soluble-fiber include oats and oat bran, legumes (peas, beans, lentils), some fruits and vegetables such as blueberries, pears, and cucumbers. Soluble fiber slows downs digestion and keeps you feeling full longer. Since it slows down the emptying of your stomach, it helps keep blood sugar balanced.

Insoluble fiber does not dissolve in water and passes through our digestive systems intact. Because it remains unchanged in its form, insoluble fiber speeds up the transit time of food in the gut, essentially "cleaning you out" by producing a laxative effect. Sources of insoluble fiber include wheat bran, whole grains, and a large variety of vegetables and fruits.

Most vegetables and fruits contain both soluble and insoluble fiber.

Some of the high-fiber foods we eat are known as prebiotics and are especially helpful because they contain a class of dietary fiber known as "inulin." Prebiotics help reverse FATflammation by helping the good and friendly bacteria in our digestive system do their jobs.

Remember, an inflamed gut increases your tendency to become overfat. Prebiotic inulins ferment in the large intestine; the end result of that fermentation process is a healthy dose of beneficial bacteria. Inulins are found in veggies such as asparagus, onions, leeks, and garlic. Two of the best sources of inulin are chicory root and yacon syrup. Note: yacon syrup is an allowed sweetener in the FATflammation-Free Diet Program. Try it to get a little extra sweetness in your life along with a healthy dose of prebiotic inulin.

New research gives us even more reason for increasing the amount of fiber (particularly inulin) we ingest every day. A recent animal study identified an antiappetite molecule that is released when we digest fiber. The study showed that mice fed a high-fat diet with added inulin ate less and gained less weight than similar mice fed a high-fat diet without inulin. Researchers then tracked the molecule through the body, showing that it ended up in the part of the brain that controls hunger.

Many of the foods in the FATflammation-Free Diet Program are high in fiber. Beans/legumes, berries, nuts, chia seeds, avocados, and leafy vegetables such as kale and collard greens are all high in fiber. Asparagus, onions, leeks, and garlic are all high in inulin, as is yacon syrup. All these foods help ensure a healthy, less inflamed gut, which leads directly to fat loss. So don't forget to eat your veggies and fruits such as berries.

Your ideal fiber goal is 30–50 grams a day. If you are not accustomed to eating fiber, do not include that much fiber without first allowing your body to become adjusted. Also don't forget to drink water. You want to keep that fiber moving through your digestive tract; you don't want to run the risk of constipation.

On the Suggested Supplement List in the appendix is a fiber supplement called glucomamman, which is a water-soluble polysaccharide and dietary fiber. I recommend this to all my clients and think it's a helpful dieting tool. You can buy this in most health stores as well as online. As mentioned earlier, the brand I use is called PGX, but many others are available. Taking a supplement will help you reach your fiber intake goal. Follow product instructions. Make sure that you take it with a full 8-ounce glass of water. The fiber absorbs the water and really does make you feel as though you have had plenty to eat. Studies have shown significant weight loss among those taking glucomannan compared to those taking a placebo.

CHAPTER 12

WEEK ONE—GETTING STARTED

"You have to get clean to get lean."

▶ Week One will immediately begin shrinking your fat cells and breaking the inflamed fat cell cycle. You will also be cleaning out your liver and helping your body detox. I've said this before, but I'm going to say it again; your liver is your number one fat-burning organ, and getting it "clean" helps it fulfill its function of burning fat. This week will also get your blood sugar back in balance so you can stop the roller coaster of blood sugar spikes and precipitous drops that lead to inflamed fat cells and FATflammation.

Week One is the most challenging and stringent of the three weeks because you will be removing a variety of foods that you are accustomed to eating, such as sugar and refined carbohydrates. Here's your mantra for the week: *You have to get clean to get lean.*

During this week, you will also be developing new habits such as drinking more water and eating three meals and two snacks daily. Within a very few days, you should begin to lose your taste for sugar and other refined carbohydrates, but if you feel hungry and have cravings—or even worry about feeling hungry and having cravings—don't forget about chromium picolinate and PGX fiber (check the supplement list starting on page 212).

The best part of Week One is that you are becoming FATflammation free! It's always such a joy for me to watch people shrink their fat cells. I love seeing them lose weight and feel great!

TRACKING FOOD SENSITIVITY—WEEK ONE

During Week One, you will be giving up all grains, including those that contain gluten. You will also be avoiding all dairy, except yogurt. This will help you rule out the possibility that you are "sensitive" to these foods. (Notes: The asterisks throughout the days' plans here indicate recipes included in the appendix. The list of optional allowed sweeteners can be found on page 228.)

WEEK ONE—DAY ONE

As Soon as You Wake Up

Drink 1 cup warm/hot lemon water.

20 Minutes Before Breakfast

Drink two (8-ounce) glasses cool/cold water.

Breakfast

Scrambled Eggs with Avocado, Sun-Dried Tomatoes, and Mushrooms*
Take your supplements.

Midmorning Snack

½ cup plain regular (2%) or unsweetened coconut yogurt mixed with ¼ cup berries (see list) and cinnamon. (See optional allowed sweeteners.)

20 Minutes Before Lunch

Drink two (8-ounce) glasses cool/cold water.

Lunch

4 ounces of wild water-packed canned salmon mixed with 1 teaspoon olive oil, onions, chopped celery, capers (optional) rolled up in coconut (or lettuce) wrap. (To make a lettuce wrap, just take one or two large leaves of romaine lettuce.)

Salad of spinach leaves mixed with red bell peppers, red onion, and
   drizzled with 1 teaspoon extra-virgin olive oil and, if desired,
   balsamic vinegar or lemon juice

Midafternoon Snack

Blanched or raw asparagus spears wrapped with 1 slice of prosciutto
   or 1 slice turkey

20 Minutes Before Dinner

Drink two (8-ounce) glasses of cool/cold water—add 1 teaspoon of
   apple cider vinegar to one glass.

Dinner

Texas Skillet Turkey Dinner*
String beans or veggie of choice (see list)
Avocado Arugula Salad with Blueberries*

WEEK ONE—DAY TWO

As Soon as You Wake Up

Drink 1 cup warm/hot lemon water.

20 Minutes Before Breakfast

Drink two (8-ounce) glasses cool/cold water.

Breakfast

Lori's Spicy Chai Smoothie*
Take your supplements.

Midmorning Snack

**2 slices lean roast beef wrapped around a veggie of your choice such as
   romaine, bell pepper, string bean, cucumber, celery, asparagus**

20 Minutes Before Lunch

Drink two (8-ounce) glasses cool/cold water.

Lunch

Tuna-Pistachio Stuffed Tomatoes*
Small salad (1–2 cups chopped greens) with ¼ cup blueberries, red onion, 1 teaspoon olive oil and, if desired, balsamic vinegar or lemon juice

Midafternoon Snack

½ cup plain regular (2%) or unsweetened coconut yogurt mixed with allowed fruit of your choice from list (See optional allowed sweeteners.)

20 Minutes Before Dinner

Drink two (8-ounce) glasses cool/cold water—one glass with 1 teaspoon of apple cider vinegar.

Dinner

4 to 6 ounces chicken (strips) stir-fried with mushrooms, onions, peppers
Spinach and Bean Sauté*

WEEK ONE—DAY THREE

As Soon as You Wake Up

Drink 1 cup warm/hot lemon water.

20 Minutes Before Breakfast

Drink two (8-ounce) glasses cool/cold water.

Breakfast

2 eggs (poached, scrambled, boiled, sunny-side up) over sautéed spinach

4 to 6 ounces low-sodium vegetable or tomato juice (If you don't like tomato-based juice, make your own green vegetable juice or eat a sliced tomato or other raw vegetables you prefer.)
Take your supplements.

Midmorning Snack

½ cup plain regular (2%) yogurt or unsweetened coconut yogurt mixed with ¼ cup of berries (see list). (See optional allowed sweeteners.)

20 Minutes Before Lunch

Drink two (8-ounce) glasses cool/cold water.

Lunch

Turkey Hummus BLT Wrap*
Small mixed watercress and spinach salad drizzled with 1 teaspoon olive oil and, if desired, balsamic vinegar or lemon juice

Midafternoon Snack

1 serving packet light tuna fish (2.6 ounces) and celery sticks (add 2 teaspoons olive oil to tuna)

20 Minutes Before Dinner

Drink two (8-ounce) glasses cool/cold water—one glass with 1 teaspoon of apple cider vinegar.

Dinner

3-Bean Beef Chili*
Oven-roasted summer and/or zucchini squash (or veggies of choice—see list)
Small salad with mixed greens with 1 teaspoon olive oil and, if desired, balsamic vinegar or lemon juice

WEEK ONE—DAY FOUR

As Soon as You Wake Up

Drink 1 cup warm/hot lemon water.

20 Minutes Before Breakfast

Drink two (8-ounce) glasses cool/cold water.

Breakfast

Omelet made with 2 whole eggs + 1 egg white, fresh basil, chopped fresh tomatoes

2 slices of Canadian bacon

4 to 6 ounces low-sodium vegetable or tomato juice (If you don't like tomato-based juice, make your own green vegetable juice or eat a sliced tomato or other raw vegetables you prefer.)

Take your supplements.

Midmorning Snack

½ cup plain regular (2%) yogurt or unsweetened coconut yogurt plus berries of choice (See optional allowed sweeteners.)

20 Minutes Before Lunch

Drink two (8-ounce) glasses cool/cold water.

Lunch

4 to 6 ounces grilled shrimp

Broccoli and cauliflower florets drizzled with ½ teaspoon olive oil

Small salad of choice (see recipes in appendix)

Midafternoon Snack

Fresh veggies of choice and 2 tablespoons of hummus

20 Minutes Before Dinner

Drink two (8-ounce) glasses cool/cold water—one glass with
1 teaspoon of apple cider vinegar.

Dinner

Ground Turkey Stuffed Peppers*
Salad with mixed greens, ¼ avocado drizzled with 1 teaspoon olive oil
  and, if desired, balsamic vinegar or lemon juice

WEEK ONE—DAY FIVE

As Soon as You Wake Up

Drink 1 cup warm/hot lemon water.

20 Minutes Before Breakfast

Drink two (8-ounce) glasses cool/cold water.

Breakfast

Berry Coconut Yogurt Smoothie*
Take your supplements.

Midmorning Snack

Hard-boiled egg and sliced tomatoes (Optional addition: Salsa)

20 Minutes Before Lunch

Drink two (8-ounce) glasses cool/cold water.

Lunch

---

4 ounces of grilled salmon over bed of veggies of choice
¼ cup mushrooms, ½ cup chopped broccoli sautéed in 1 tablespoon
  coconut oil

Midafternoon Snack

5 macadamia nuts and a kiwi

20 Minutes Before Dinner

Drink two (8-ounce) glasses cool/cold water—add 1 teaspoon apple cider vinegar to one glass.

Dinner

Chicken Marinara*
Steamed asparagus
Salad with 1 cup chopped spinach, ¼ cup cannellini beans, sliced red onion, drizzled with 1 teaspoon olive oil and, if desired, balsamic vinegar or lemon juice

WEEK ONE—DAY SIX

As Soon as You Wake Up

Drink 1 cup warm/hot lemon water.

20 Minutes Before Breakfast

Drink two (8-ounce) glasses cool/cold water.

Breakfast

Coconut Chocolate Milk Smoothie*
Take your supplements.

Midmorning Snack

½ cup plain regular (2%) or unsweetened coconut yogurt and 5 almonds. (See optional sweeteners.)

20 Minutes Before Lunch

Drink two (8-ounce) glasses cool/cold water.

Lunch

---

4 to 6 ounces sardines (water packed)

Spinach salad with sliced red onion and red pepper drizzled with 1 teaspoon macadamia nut oil and, if desired, balsamic vinegar or lemon juice

Midafternoon Snack

¼ cup Hummus Dip* or Lentil Dip* with veggie of choice

20 Minutes Before Dinner

Drink two (8-ounce) glasses cool/cold water—add 1 teaspoon apple cider vinegar to one glass.

Dinner

Chicken strips (4 to 6 ounces), 1 tablespoon chopped walnuts, snow peas, and water chestnuts stir-fried in 2 tablespoons macadamia oil

½ baked sweet potato (medium sized) with 1 teaspoon coconut oil (reserve other half potato for tomorrow's breakfast)

Steamed broccoli

Small mixed green salad with 1 teaspoon olive oil and, if desired, balsamic vinegar or lemon juice

WEEK ONE—DAY SEVEN

As Soon as You Wake Up

Drink 1 cup warm/hot lemon water.

20 Minutes Before Breakfast

Drink two (8-ounce) glasses cool/cold water.

Breakfast

---

2 eggs (soft-boiled, poached, or scrambled)

½ cup sweet potato hash (Cut up sweet potato left over from dinner and sauté quickly in 1 tablespoon coconut oil.)

Take your supplements.

Midmorning Snack

½ cup plain regular (2%) or unsweetened coconut yogurt and 1 kiwi (See optional allowed sweeteners.)

20 Minutes Before Lunch

Drink two (8-ounce) glasses cool/cold water.

Lunch

---

4 ounces of canned salmon mixed with 1 teaspoon olive oil.

Arugula salad with ¼ cup of garbanzo beans, ¼ cup blueberries, lightly drizzled with 1 teaspoon olive oil and, if desired, balsamic vinegar or lemon juice

Midafternoon Snack

---

2 slices deli chicken wrapped around jicama, celery, and/or asparagus

5 raw walnuts

20 Minutes Before Dinner

Drink two (8-ounce) glasses cool/cold water—one glass with 1 teaspoon of apple cider vinegar.

Dinner

Lentil and Turkey Sausage Soup*

Salad with mixed greens, red, yellow, and green bell peppers sprinkled with blueberries and drizzled with 1 teaspoon macadamia nut oil and balsamic vinegar or lemon juice

Asparagus drizzled with lemon

CHAPTER 13

WEEK TWO—GETTING AHEAD

"I did it! I finished the first week. Dr. Lori told me that
the first few days I would be detoxing because I was
withdrawing from all the sugar and processed food I was
accustomed to eating and I might feel a little crummy. It
actually wasn't that bad. By day four I felt fine and my
cravings had actually pretty much disappeared."

—LAURA

▶ Congratulations! You have completed seven days of detox to get "clean" and reset your metabolism. You have "kicked" sugar to the curb and reduced the excess insulin that was creating FATflammation. Your liver is better able to do its fat-burning work; your blood sugar is more balanced; your digestive tract is less inflamed. The yogurt you have been eating and the probiotics you have been taking have made the "good bugs" (bacteria) in your gut much happier, which will help promote further weight loss. By Week Two, you shouldn't be experiencing hunger or cravings. Best of all, your fat cells are shrinking and you should be starting to see weight loss. You should also have more energy and this is just the beginning. Remember, you are becoming FATflammation Free.

TRACKING ANY FOOD SENSITIVITIES

During Week One, you stopped eating all grains and dairy except for yogurt. During Week Two, you will continue to avoid grains that include gluten.

However, you will be adding gluten-free whole grains such as brown rice. You will also begin to eat other dairy products, such as cheese. If you eat dairy and start to experience any of the symptoms associated with food sensitivity such as bloating, diarrhea, digestive upset, nasal congestion, headaches, or rashes, this lets you know that you are sensitive to dairy and need to start substituting nondairy foods.

WEEK TWO—DAY ONE

As Soon as You Wake Up

Drink 1 cup warm/hot lemon water.

20 Minutes Before Breakfast

Drink two (8-ounce) glasses cool/cold water.

Breakfast

Spinach, Feta Cheese, and Mushroom Omelet*
4 to 6 ounces low-sodium vegetable or tomato juice (If you don't like tomato-based juice, make your own green vegetable juice or eat a sliced tomato or other raw vegetables you prefer.)
Take your supplements.

Midmorning Snack

½ cup plain regular (2%) or unsweetened coconut yogurt mixed with ⅓ cup of blueberries and cinnamon to taste. (See optional allowed sweeteners.)

20 Minutes Before Lunch

Drink two (8-ounce) glasses cool/cold water.

Lunch

Chicken Nuggets*

Arugula, red onion, and blueberry salad drizzled with 1 teaspoon olive
oil and, if desired, balsamic vinegar or lemon juice
Veggie of choice

Midafternoon Snack

2 slices roast beef wrapped around ¼ avocado, sliced

20 Minutes Before Dinner

Drink two (8-ounce) glasses cool/cold water—one glass with
1 teaspoon of apple cider vinegar.

Dinner

Almond-Crusted Cod*
Kale and Mashed Avocado Salad*
Choice of any veggie

WEEK TWO—DAY TWO

As Soon as You Wake Up

Drink 1 cup warm/hot lemon water.

20 Minutes Before Breakfast

Drink two (8-ounce) glasses cool/cold water.

Breakfast

1 serving oatmeal (steel-cut) (with 2 tablespoons whey, ⅛ teaspoon
each of cinnamon, ginger, and nutmeg) and almond milk
Take your supplements.

Midmorning Snack

½ cup plain regular (2%) or unsweetened coconut yogurt and ½ apple
for dipping (See optional allowed sweeteners.)

20 Minutes Before Lunch

Drink two (8-ounce) glasses cool/cold water.

Lunch

Julie's Greek Chicken Soup with Brown Rice*

Chopped green salad (romaine, kale, spinach, arugula)

Midafternoon Snack

5 large Taro chips with ¼ cup Hummus Dip* (See dip recipes in appendix.)

20 Minutes Before Dinner

Drink two (8-ounce) glasses cool/cold water—one glass with 1 teaspoon of apple cider vinegar.

Dinner

Hot Garlic Shrimp*

½ cup cooked wild or brown rice

Your choice of veggies

WEEK TWO—DAY THREE

As Soon as You Wake Up

Drink 1 cup warm/hot lemon water.

20 Minutes Before Breakfast

Drink two (8-ounce) glasses cool/cold water.

Breakfast

Lori's Luscious Smoothie*

Take your supplements.

Midmorning Snack

½ cup plain regular (2%) or unsweetened coconut yogurt mixed with fresh or defrosted frozen raspberries (See optional allowed sweeteners.)

20 Minutes Before Lunch

Drink two (8-ounce) glasses cool/cold water.

Lunch

Open-Face Tuna Sandwich Melt*
Sliced tomato

Midafternoon Snack

Endive or romaine stuffed with ¼ cup of lentil or hummus dip

20 Minutes Before Dinner

Drink two (8-ounce) glasses cool/cold water—one glass with 1 teaspoon of apple cider vinegar.

Dinner

Bean Soup with Smoked Turkey Sausage*
Veggie of choice
Small Spinach Salad with Red Bell Peppers and Red Onions*

WEEK TWO—DAY FOUR

As Soon as You Wake Up

Drink 1 cup warm/hot lemon water.

20 Minutes Before Breakfast

Drink two (8-ounce) glasses cool/cold water.

Breakfast

Protein Pancakes*
¼ cup sliced strawberries
Take your supplements.

Midmorning Snack

**½ cup plain (2%) or coconut yogurt with ¼ cup blueberries
and 1 teaspoon added chia seeds (See list of optional allowed
sweeteners.)**

20 Minutes Before Lunch

Drink two (8-ounce) glasses cool/cold water.

Lunch

Salmon Burger on a Bed of Mixed Baby Greens*
Veggie of choice

Midafternoon Snack

---

1 cup low-sodium lentil soup

20 Minutes Before Dinner

**Drink two (8-ounce) glasses cool/cold water—one glass with
1 teaspoon of apple cider vinegar.**

Dinner

---

4 to 6 ounces of grilled chicken breast
½ cup cooked brown rice with 1 teaspoon butter
Sliced tomatoes drizzled with 1 teaspoon olive oil
Veggie of choice

WEEK TWO—DAY FIVE

As Soon as You Wake Up

Drink 1 cup warm/hot lemon water.

20 Minutes Before Breakfast

Drink two (8-ounce) glasses cool/cold water.

Breakfast

2 eggs (poached, scrambled, sunny side up, or boiled)
2 turkey sausage links
4 to 6 ounces low-sodium vegetable or tomato juice (If you don't like tomato-based juice, make your own green vegetable juice or eat a sliced tomato or other raw vegetables you prefer.)
Take your supplements.

Midmorning Snack

½ cup plain regular (2%) or unsweetened coconut yogurt mixed with ¼ cup fresh or defrosted berries. (See optional allowed sweeteners.)

20 Minutes Before Lunch

Drink two glasses (8-ounce) cool/cold water.

Lunch

Shrimp and Veggie Stir-Fry*
½ cup brown rice or quinoa
Small green salad with 1 teaspoon olive oil and, if desired, balsamic vinegar or lemon juice

Midafternoon Snack

½ apple with 1 ounce of cheddar cheese

20 Minutes Before Dinner

Drink two (8-ounce) glasses cool/cold water—one glass with 1 teaspoon of apple cider vinegar.

Dinner

"Pasta" and Turkey Marinara Sauce*
Veggie of choice

WEEK TWO—DAY SIX

As Soon as You Wake Up

Drink 1 cup warm/hot lemon water.

20 Minutes Before Breakfast

Drink two (8-ounce) glasses cool/cold water.

Breakfast

2 whole eggs scrambled with spinach, plus ¼ avocado, sliced, with ½ gluten-free pita (salsa optional)
½ grapefruit
Take your supplements.

Midmorning Snack

½ cup plain regular (2%) or unsweetened coconut yogurt with ¼ cup berries of choice. (See optional allowed sweeteners.)

20 Minutes Before Lunch

Drink two (8-ounce) glasses cool/cold water.

Lunch

Turkey Burger Avocado Wrap*
Veggie of choice

Midafternoon Snack

Veggie sticks with 2 tablespoons almond butter

20 Minutes Before Dinner

Drink two (8-ounce) glasses cool/cold water—one glass with 1 teaspoon of apple cider vinegar.

Dinner

Prosciutto-Wrapped Cod*
Baked ½ sweet potato
Veggie of choice
Small salad of choice (see recipes in appendix)

WEEK TWO—DAY SEVEN

As Soon as You Wake Up

Drink 1 cup warm/hot lemon water.

20 Minutes Before Breakfast

Drink two (8-ounce) glasses cool/cold water.

Breakfast

½ toasted gluten-free sprouted English muffin (with 1 teaspoon butter)
½ cup cottage cheese mixed with 1 teaspoon chia seeds
4 to 6 ounces low-sodium vegetable or tomato juice (If you don't like tomato-based juice, make your own green vegetable juice or eat a sliced tomato or other raw vegetables you prefer.)
Take your supplements.

Midmorning Snack

Berry Yogurt Parfait*

20 Minutes Before Lunch

Drink two (8-ounce) glasses cool/cold water.

Lunch

Crunchy Mozzarella Salmon Melt*
Small spinach salad of your choice (see recipes in appendix)

Midafternoon Snack

---

2 roasted asparagus spears each wrapped in 1 small slice of prosciutto

20 Minutes Before Dinner

**Drink two (8-ounce) glasses cool/cold water—one glass with
1 teaspoon of apple cider vinegar.**

Dinner

---

4 to 6 ounces broiled sirloin steak (preferably grass fed)
½ cup cooked wild rice, quinoa, or brown rice
Steamed veggie of choice with 1 teaspoon olive oil
Small salad of your choice (see recipes on page 257)

CHAPTER 14

WEEK THREE—GAINING MASTERY

*"I can't believe how much weight I've lost. I've lost
more than ten pounds. My skin looks better. I'm even
sleeping better. I absolutely do not crave sugar or carbs,
and I have more energy than I've had in years."*
—CATHY

▶ YOU are awesome! You really should be proud of yourself for doing what you had to do to get control of those fat cells! By now, you have concrete proof that it is not willpower or counting points or calories that create weight loss. You are losing weight because you are eating the right foods and have stopped eating the foods that create FATflammation!

Week Three is about gaining control or mastery of what you've learned thus far. In this week, you will continue to eat clean and balance omega-3/omega-6 fats. By now, you should have pretty much conquered your addiction to sugar and refined carbs. Just don't slip back!

TRACKING ANY FOOD SENSITIVITIES

In Week Three, you will be adding wheat (which contains gluten) back into your diet. If you eat wheat and experience any of the symptoms associated with food sensitivity such as bloating, diarrhea, digestive upset, nasal congestion, headaches, or rashes, this lets you know that you are sensitive to gluten and are one of those people who needs to remove all gluten products from your diet.

WEEK THREE—DAY ONE

As Soon as You Wake Up

Drink 1 cup warm/hot lemon water.

20 minutes before breakfast

Drink two (8-ounce) glasses cool/cold water.

Breakfast

**1 serving oatmeal (steel-cut) (with 2 tablespoons whey and
⅛ teaspoon each of cinnamon and nutmeg) and almond milk,
¼ cup sliced fresh or unsweetened frozen strawberries
Take your supplements.**

Midmorning Snack

**½ cup plain regular (2%) or unsweetened coconut yogurt with fresh
or frozen berries of choice (See optional allowed sweeteners.)**

20 Minutes Before Lunch

Drink two (8-ounce) glasses cool/cold water.

Lunch

**4 ounces baked wild salmon with dill
Parmesan-Crusted Zucchini Medallions* (can be made in advance)
Baby Arugula, Avocado, and Tomato Salad***

Midafternoon Snack

**Deviled Hummus Egg* with cut-up green veggie sticks (such as
zucchini, celery, green pepper)**

20 Minutes Before Dinner

**Drink two (8-ounce) glasses cool/cold water—one glass with
1 teaspoon of apple cider vinegar.**

Dinner

Grilled 4- to 6-ounce turkey burger with 1 thin slice of cheese in low-carb whole-grain wrap

½ cup cooked brown rice

Small Salad of Mixed Baby Greens and Bell Peppers*

WEEK THREE—DAY TWO

As Soon as You Wake Up

Drink 1 cup warm/hot lemon water.

20 Minutes Before Breakfast

Drink two (8-ounce) glasses cool/cold water.

Breakfast

2 eggs any style

2 slices of turkey bacon

4 to 6 ounces low-sodium vegetable or tomato juice (If you don't like tomato-based juice, make your own green vegetable juice or eat a sliced tomato or other raw vegetables you prefer.)

Take your supplements.

Midmorning Snack

½ cup plain regular (2%) or unsweetened coconut yogurt with blueberries (See optional allowed sweeteners.)

20 Minutes Before Lunch

Drink two (8-ounce) glasses cool/cold water.

Lunch

Chicken Salad in Pita Pocket*

Small Chopped Romaine Salad*

Midafternoon Snack

½ apple, sliced and smeared with 1 tablespoon coconut, almond, or peanut butter

20 Minutes Before Dinner

Drink two (8-ounce) glasses cool/cold water.

Dinner

Penne Pasta with Shrimp and Sausage*
Veggie of choice
Small Arugula and Butter Lettuce Salad*

WEEK THREE—DAY THREE

As Soon as You Wake Up

Drink 1 cup warm/hot lemon water.

20 Minutes Before Breakfast

Drink two (8-ounce) glasses cool/cold water.

Breakfast

½ whole-grain-sprouted pita, 2 scrambled eggs, ¼ sliced avocado, ½ roasted or fresh green pepper (optional)

4 to 6 ounces low-sodium vegetable or tomato juice (If you don't like tomato-based juice, make your own green vegetable juice or eat a sliced tomato or other raw vegetables you prefer.)

Take your supplements.

Midmorning Snack

¼ cup of berries, 1 tablespoon chopped walnut mixed in ½ cup plain regular (2%) or unsweetened coconut yogurt or low-fat ricotta cheese (See optional allowed sweeteners.)

20 Minutes Before Lunch

Drink two (8-ounce) glasses cool/cold water.

Lunch

Salad Nicoise*

Midafternoon Snack

2 thin slices of deli turkey and ½ pear

20 Minutes Before Dinner

Drink two (8-ounce) glasses cool/cold water—one glass with
1 teaspoon of apple cider vinegar.

Dinner

Walnut Pesto Cod*
½ cup of cooked quinoa
Veggie of choice
Small salad of your choice (see recipes in appendix)

WEEK THREE—DAY FOUR

As Soon as You Wake Up

Drink 1 cup warm/hot lemon water.

20 Minutes Before Breakfast

Drink two (8 oz) glasses cool/cold water.

Breakfast

Berry Ginger Smoothie*
Take your supplements.

Midmorning Snack

   1 hard-boiled egg

   1 small tomato or handful of grape tomatoes

20 Minutes Before Lunch

   Drink two (8-ounce) glasses cool/cold water.

Lunch

   4 ounces roasted chicken breast

   ½ cup cooked brown rice

   Steamed baby kale drizzled with 1 teaspoon olive oil

Midafternoon Snack

   ½ cup plain regular (2%) or unsweetened coconut yogurt with
     ¼ cup chopped apple (See optional allowed sweeteners.)

20 Minutes Before Dinner

   Drink two (8-ounce) glasses cool/cold water—one glass with
     1 teaspoon of apple cider vinegar.

Dinner

   Sesame Fish*

   ½ cup cooked brown rice or ½ cup garbanzo beans

   Veggie of choice

   Salad of choice (see appendix recipes)

WEEK THREE—DAY FIVE

As Soon as You Wake Up

   Drink 1 cup warm/hot lemon water.

20 Minutes Before Breakfast

   Drink two (8-ounce) glasses cool/cold water.

Breakfast

Sausage, Spinach, and Cheese Egg Muffins*

4 to 6 ounces low-sodium vegetable or tomato juice (If you don't like tomato-based juice, make your own green vegetable juice or eat a sliced tomato or other raw vegetables you prefer.)

Take your supplements.

Midmorning Snack

½ cup plain regular (2%) plain or unsweetened coconut yogurt and ¼ cup fresh or defrosted strawberries (See optional allowed sweeteners.)

20 Minutes Before Lunch

Drink two (8-ounce) glasses cool/cold water.

Lunch

4-ounce lean grilled beef patty (preferably grass fed) on a bed of baby greens, drizzled with 1 teaspoon olive oil and topped with handful of grape tomatoes, ¼ sliced avocado, and pico de gallo or salsa (optional)

Midafternoon Snack

Celery sticks with 1 tablespoon of peanut butter or nut butter of choice

20 Minutes Before Dinner

Drink two (8-ounce) glasses cool/cold water—one glass with 1 teaspoon of apple cider vinegar.

Dinner

Halibut Tacos*
Sautéed Spicy Green Beans*
Small Chopped Romaine Salad*

WEEK THREE—DAY SIX

As Soon as You Wake Up

Drink 1 cup warm/hot lemon water.

20 Minutes Before Breakfast

Drink two (8-ounce) glasses cool/cold water.

Breakfast

FATflammation-Free Smoothie*
Take your supplements.

Midmorning Snack

1 kiwi and 5 macadamia nuts

20 Minutes Before Lunch

Drink two (8-ounce) glasses cool/cold water.

Lunch

Chicken and Wild Rice Soup*
**1 small salad with ½ small avocado drizzled with 1 teaspoon olive oil
    and lemon juice**

Midafternoon Snack

Black Bean Dip* with fresh veggies

20 Minutes Before Dinner

**Drink two (8-ounce) glasses cool/cold water—one glass with
    1 teaspoon of apple cider vinegar.**

Dinner

Roast Turkey Thighs with Herbs*
Steamed broccoli stalks drizzled with 1 tablespoon macadamia nut oil
   and lemon juice
½ cup cooked brown rice
Small green salad of choice (see appendix recipes)

WEEK THREE—DAY SEVEN

As Soon as You Wake Up

Drink 1 cup warm/hot lemon water.

20 Minutes Before Breakfast

Drink two (8-ounce) glasses cool/cold water.

Breakfast

Quick Breakfast Burritos*
4 to 6 ounces low-sodium vegetable or tomato juice (If you don't like
   tomato-based juice, make your own green vegetable juice or eat a
   sliced tomato or other raw vegetable you prefer.)
Take your supplements.

Midmorning Snack

½ cup plain regular (2%) or unsweetened coconut yogurt mixed with
   1 teaspoon chia seeds and ¼ cup fresh or unsweetened frozen
   berries (See optional allowed sweeteners.)

20 Minutes Before Lunch

Drink two (8-ounce) glasses cool/cold water.

Lunch

Quick Black Bean Burger*
Steamed greens

Midafternoon Snack

2 thin slices of turkey with 2 veggie stalks (such as asparagus, zucchini, celery, green pepper)
5 macadamia nuts

20 Minutes Before Dinner

Drink two (8-ounce) glasses cool/cold water—one glass with 1 teaspoon of apple cider vinegar.

Dinner

Sautéed Garlic Sea Scallops*
½ cup cooked quinoa, wild rice, or brown rice
Veggie of choice
Small Chopped Kale Salad*

PART FOUR

FATFLAMMATION
FREE
FOREVER!

CHAPTER 15

THE FATFLAMMATION-FREE LIFESTYLE

"My life really has changed. I don't feel powerless. I'm in control of what I eat and I don't feel as though I'm being controlled by food. I finally feel as though I'm at a place where I want to exercise, and I feel as though exercise is a real part of my life. As I see the weight coming off, I feel confident that I will be able to keep doing this. I'm really comfortable with my new lifestyle."

—SUSAN

▶ Congratulations! You did the work and completed all three weeks of the FATflammation-Free Diet Program. You deserve a great deal of applause. So stop for a moment and acknowledge your achievements. Think about all you accomplished: instead of bemoaning your issues with weight, you took control of your life. You took action! This is fabulous and wonderful. I know there have been challenges, but you have been able to move through them and are now seeing the positive changes you created. Yes, you did this, and now you know how powerful you can be.

The changes you have already made will have an enormous impact on the way you live and how you feel. But change, as you know, doesn't happen overnight. That's why you have to start preparing for everything you will need to do so that you can continue forward until you reach your weight-loss goal. A karate student, who has just earned a well-deserved black belt, is now recognized as a master, but he/she also knows that mastery involves continuous commitment and work. You too are a master now and, in a sense, have a "black belt" in reversing FATflammation. Being able to continue forward on this path has everything to do with staying motivated and being willing to do the necessary work. Because of all the work you have done, you know the basic principles of the FATflammation-Free Diet Program, and you have established some strong habits that will serve you well.

You know what causes FATflammation, but let's go through the list again. This is what you need to avoid.

Dehydration (even mild)
Sugar and artificial sweeteners
High-fructose corn syrup
Trans fats
Refined grains
**Foods high in omega-6 oils (including oils such as corn, peanut,
     soy, safflower, and sunflower)**
Foods to which you are allergic or have a specific sensitivity
Too much stress
Imbalanced digestive bacteria
Not enough sleep
Too little exercise

You know how to fight FAT*flammation*. This is what you need to do.

Drink more water.
Add protein to every meal and snack.
Include cultured foods and probiotics daily.
**Increase your daily intake of omega-3 fatty acids (found in
     cold-water fish and omega-3 supplements).**
**Use only healthy oils such as olive oil, coconut oil, and
     macadamia nut oil.**
Eat more fiber.
**Mind your micronutrients (make certain you are getting all the
     minerals, vitamins and phytonutrients that you need).**
Eliminate foods to which you might be allergic or sensitive.

Reduce your stress.
Get more sleep.
Exercise.

By now you are an expert in the daily routine, but let's review it one more time.

EACH DAY

As soon as you wake up, drink a cup of lemon water (juice of ½ lemon in hot/warm water)

Drink two (8-ounce) glasses of water before breakfast.
Eat breakfast.
Take your supplements.
Have a midmorning snack.
Drink two (8-ounce) glasses of water before lunch.
Eat lunch.
Have a midafternoon snack.
Drink two (8-ounce) glasses of water, one with 1 teaspoon cider
    vinegar before dinner.
Eat dinner.

AVOID PORTION DISTORTION

Another example of mindless eating has to do with portion size. Over the years, portion sizes in this country have become larger and larger, and we have all become accustomed to chowing down on portions that are way larger than anything that could be thought of as reasonable or healthy. According to the U.S. Department of Health and Human Services, twenty years ago, two slices of pepperoni pizza had 500 calories. And in all probability that pizza was made using olive oil and fresh cheese. And the sauce, made from Grandma's recipe featured "a small pinch," not large amounts, of sugar or, even worse, HFCS. Today, two slices is about 850 calories. And who knows precisely what we are eating. Twenty years ago, the average-size portion of pasta was one cup of pasta and three meatballs, and it was 500 calories. Today, the average-size portion of pasta comes to two cups and by the time you add in all the sauce and meat, the calories clock in at 1,025. These are the sizes most people have come to expect. Today, the average person looking at a one-cup serving of pasta tends to think it is skimpy.

Here is something to keep in mind: your stomach is only about the size of your fist. It stretches to accommodate the food you eat. . . . And we don't want it to stretch too far, do we?

MEASURED PORTION SIZES FOR ONE SERVING

Here are some portion sizes to help you remember how much you should be eating.

Protein = 4–6 ounces
Nonstarchy vegetables = unlimited
Starchy vegetables = ½ cup cooked, ½ sweet potato
Whole grains = ½ cup cooked
Beans/legumes = ½ cup cooked
Fruit = one medium piece, ½ cup berries or diced fruit
Nuts and seeds = ¼ cup or small shallow handful

FATFLAMMATION-FREE MEAL

When people ask me how much they should be eating at a meal, I tell them about what I call the "FATflammation-Free Meal."

Using a nine-inch plate, fill one-quarter with lean protein; fill one-quarter with starchy veggies or beans/legumes; fill one-half with nonstarchy veggies.

Add a small green salad. Include 1 to 2 tablespoons of healthy fat (olive oil, coconut oil, macadamia nut oil) per meal, including the cooking oil and oil on vegetables and salad.

"WILL I EVER BE ABLE TO EAT DESSERT AGAIN?"

This is a question that I hear all the time. People want to know whether they will ever again be able to indulge in refined carbohydrates. This is a fair question. Before I answer, I want to assure you that I am certainly not perfect in terms of all my food choices, and I don't expect you to be perfect either. However, I do think you need to be very conscientious about your diet. Of course there will be times when you lapse and eat something we all know you shouldn't be eating. We all do it occasionally. What you need to know is that if you do "slip" and overeat, you have to take it for what it is: a solitary episode and not the end of your path to staying FATflammation Free. Just acknowledge what happened, brush yourself off, and get back on track.

HANDLING FOOD TEMPTATION

So let's say you are at a party, and somebody hands you a plate that contains a piece of pie or a slice of strawberry shortcake or a chocolate brownie—and you don't think you can resist the temptation. What do you do? I suggest that you follow the "Three Bite Rule." Have one bite to see what it tastes like. The second bite confirms what you knew from the first bite. By the third bite, you know what it tastes like so at least part of the "thrill" is gone. Have those three bites and no more. You can probably get away with the three-bite rule once a week without it doing serious damage to your weight goals.

Another way of handling food temptation is to slow down and take only one mindful bite. Appreciate every nanosecond that it is in your mouth. Feel, taste, savor your one wonderful bite. Chew it very, very slowly and be completely aware of what you are experiencing. You've had one extraordinary bite. But, with even one bite, realize you need to limit this kind of indulgence because we know that once we start eating sugar and refined carbohydrates, they are addictive and it becomes more and more impossible to stop.

TIPS TO KEEP YOU STRONG AND FATFLAMMATION FREE

I know that you have the resources within you to reach and maintain your weight-loss goals. Here are some tips to help you stay focused and committed.

▶ Plan ahead. This is essential. Plan your meals, write your grocery list, do your shopping, then prepare your meals and snacks ahead of time. Knowing what you are going to be eating—and when—will help you stay in control.

▶ Absolutely do not walk into the supermarket or grocery store unprepared. Know what you want to buy before you get there. Do not allow for any spur-of-the-moment impulse purchases of foods that contribute to FATflammation. Have a prepared mantra that you repeat to yourself when you walk past one of your trigger foods. As you pass near the chocolates or the raisins or the packaged macaroni and cheese, think *I choose not to eat that because* . . . then repeat your goal to yourself. Make sure your goal occupies a more important place in your head than those chocolate chip cookies. Remember, you can do this.

▶ Take your lunches and snacks to work. You are in control and you don't want to be at the mercy of your environment.

▶ Be prepared for challenges. If you have come this far, then you know that you can overcome obstacles and challenges. Expect them to happen. There will be days when you will be tempted to fall back to old patterns. When this happens, think about how crummy you are going to feel if you do this. There will be days when everybody around you is eating something you shouldn't be eating. If you expect challenges, you can prepare yourself to be strong and keep to your commitment.

▶ If you do have a slipup and make some bad food choices, let go of your guilt. Guilt is not your friend. I've had clients who became so guilty about a spree of overeating that their first impulse was to give up and throw the baby out with the bathwater. However, once they calmed down and understood that the slipups did not undo their progress, they were able to get right back on track. So can you. So kick guilt to the curb and get back on the FATflammation-Free Train.

▶ Make sure you have identified your trigger foods and situations. Keep those foods out of your life and focus only on foods that reverse in FATflammation. Surround yourself with these foods. Have them available in all the places where you spend time.

▶ To improve your chances of success and double your weight loss, journal, journal, journal. Tracking what you are eating and what you are feeling will reap huge dividends.

▶ Read labels carefully. Do not allow any of the **FATflammation Four** back into your life—ever. That means no more sugar, refined grains, HFCS, or artificial sweeteners.

▶ Stay hydrated. Drink water throughout the day. Remember that the brain confuses thirst with hunger. If you think you want something to eat, have a glass of water first. Never forget that when your cells are deprived of water, cellular function—including metabolism—slows down.

▶ Whenever you have a chance, move your body. Our bodies were meant to move. If nothing else, just stand up and walk around the room or down the hall. Move your arms even if you do it at your desk when nobody is looking. Do a few leg lifts. Just keep moving. Research shows that simply moving the body by fidgeting will reap weight-loss rewards for you down the road. If you have a desk job, get up every thirty minutes. Walk around or do leg lifts or squats right there. Ten squats or leg lifts shouldn't take more than ten seconds. It all adds up.

▶ Schedule regular exercise. Choose days and times you know you will most likely keep and honor these appointments with yourself as you would a doctor's appointment. Exercise + Moving = Healthy and Fit. Always remember your "why," the reason why you wanted weight loss in the first place. Capture and relive your motivation at the beginning when your motivation was brand-new.

▶ Take your supplements. This can make a huge difference in your weight loss. Many diets fail because they don't add the layer of support that can be found in supplements. The supplements needed to reduce FATflammation are a key component to your success.

▶ Increase the amount of omega-3 in your diet by eating fish and seafood high in omega-3 and taking an omega-3 supplement.

▶ Reduce the levels of omega-6 in your diet by avoiding omega-6 seed and vegetable oils such as corn, soy, peanut, sunflower, safflower, and canola.

▶ If, during one of your weekly weighing sessions, you notice that weight is beginning to creep back up, even by as little as three pounds, immediately resume Week One.

▶ Take care of your gut. Take probiotics, and don't forget to eat food that contains prebiotics.

▶ Remember to eat lots of fiber in the form of nonstarchy veggies. Also take the fiber supplement I recommend.

▶ Calm down and practice mindfulness whenever possible. Slow down your thinking and savor the moment. Slow down your eating and savor the food. Both will reduce levels of stress. New research shows that slowing down your eating will allow your brain to receive the signal that you have had enough to eat.

CHAPTER 16

IT TAKES MORE THAN A DIET

"If you're not gonna go all the way, why go at all?"
—FOOTBALL STAR JOE NAMATH

▶ People who consult with me about their issues with "fat" are often looking for a magic bullet—one secret magical tip. I always tell them that getting rid of FATflammation involves a combination of factors. Yes, everyone who gives up sugar and refined carbohydrates will almost automatically start losing weight. Yes, adding protein to every snack and meal will help boost your metabolism. So will drinking more water. Up your intake of omega-3 fatty acids, and yes, you will start losing weight. Start doing good things for yourself by being aware of your digestive health and taking probiotics. Yep, weight loss. But reaching your goal and being FATflammation Free for life really has to do with all the factors in your life, including lifestyle issues. If you are regularly stressed to the max, not getting enough sleep, and forgetting to exercise, FATflammation is going to find its way back into your life. If you want to lose all the weight you want to lose and look the way you want to look, you have to go all the way and take on all the issues that contribute to FATflammation. Here are some ideas to help you do this.

CONFRONT YOUR STRESS

Chronic stress creates inflamed fat cells. The adrenal glands (located on the top of each kidney) are responsible for both adrenaline and cortisol, the hormone most closely associated with stress. Cortisol helps make us FAT, and it helps keep us FAT. When emotional/psychological stress is chronic, for example, cortisol sends fat to the cells in your abdominal area. Here's the kicker: as fat increases in the abdominal area, cortisol increases. In fact, as much as four times as much cortisol is produced from the deeper fat tissues in the abdominal area. Fat cells tend to increase in size because of this. This is FATflammation in action.

Cortisol also tends to increase our appetite for sugary foods. When we are emotionally stressed by life's ups and downs, many of us tend to turn to excess sugar or carbohydrates such as candy or cake. Chronic stress helps perpetuate an endless dysfunctional cycle of increased appetite, hunger, and cravings. When stress becomes chronic, cortisol responds by becoming a source of chronic inflammation.

Try Some Deep Breathing to Relieve Stress

Deep breathing really can help you deal with some of your chronic stress. When I first talk to my clients about breathing exercises, I know they don't really believe me and tend to ignore what I'm saying. I'll say the same thing to you that I say to them: "Just try it and see if you don't feel better."

Here is a very simple deep breathing exercise known as "tactical breathing." This technique, which has the power to stop your stress responses in their tracks, is the same type of deep breathing used by the military and especially our Special Forces under actual attack in combat situations. Feelings of stress and anxiety can appear in a variety of modern situations that have little to do with actual combat. When we feel stressed, our breathing tends to become shallow; sometimes we actually find ourselves holding our breath. In my experience, this "tactical breathing" exercise can get immediate results even in the most stressful and demanding situations.

Here's the method:

Slow down and breathe in through your nose for a count of four.

1, 2, 3, 4

Hold for a count of four.

1, 2, 3, 4

Exhale through your mouth for a count of four.

1, 2, 3, 4

Hold it for a count of four.

1, 2, 3, 4

Now repeat.

Do this as often as necessary.

Life Force Breathing

Another type of deep breathing, known in yoga as pranayama (life force) breathing, can do wonders for stress reduction as well as your immune system. Life force breathing is done from the diaphragm. The goal of this kind of breathing is to fill your lungs in a slow deliberate way. You'll know you are doing it right when you stomach starts protruding. Most of us are not breathing correctly. We tend to take short, shallow, fast breaths. This kind of breathing happens when we are under stress or our emotions are getting the best of us. Then, we continue to breathe this way all the time. It becomes a deeply ingrained habit that we do all the time.

There are several different ways to practice deep breathing. As long as you are truly breathing throughout your lungs and your diaphragm is expanding, then you are doing it right.

Start by lying down in a prone position on your back. Place your hands over your stomach so you notice whether your stomach is rising. When you breathe, imagine that your lungs are like an accordion with one end attached to your upper chest and the other going down to the area of your lower belly. Breathe in through your nose. Do you notice your stomach rising?

Still in the prone position, start this exercise by breathing in through your nose and out through your mouth.

Breathe in through your nose to the count of five.

1, 2, 3, 4, 5

Hold for a count of five.

1, .2, 3, 4, 5

Breathe out through your mouth to the count of five.

1, 2, 3, 4, 5

As you are breathing out, be aware of the breath gently leaving your body and feel the stress leave with every exhale.

As your diaphragm grows stronger and your lungs expand, you will be able to take in more breath. Work your way up gradually and try to go to a count of ten (or even more). Eventually you will be able to practice life force breathing without being in a prone position. In fact, it will become a natural habit, and your breathing will have changed back to what nature intended.

Work at Getting More Sleep

Could your problems with sleep be contributing to your problems with FAT-flammation? Science now says yes and points to a clear connection between chronic lack of sleep and weight gain and obesity. It's all about hormones: insufficient sleep translates into reduced insulin sensitivity, high blood sugar, elevated cortisol, increased levels of the hunger hormone ghrelin, and decreased levels of leptin, the hormone that tells you to stop eating. That sounds like a recipe for inflamed fat cells, doesn't it?

We need about seven hours of sleep a night on average. It is okay to occasionally miss out on sleep, but when it becomes chronic, you set yourself up for weight gain.

I have compiled a list of tips to help you achieve night after night of quality sleep. Give them a try. No two people are alike and thus one tip may work better for one person and not at all for another. If you find that you are still not sleeping well, I encourage you to see your doctor for more guidance.

General Tips

▶ Make sleep a priority in your life.
▶ Get some sunlight early in the day to help set your circadian rhythm.
▶ Be sure that your sleeping room is *very* dark to trigger the sleep hormone melatonin. If it isn't, consider wearing an eye mask.
▶ Is the temperature cool enough? Studies show that we sleep better in temperatures that are lower than those we are accustomed to during the day.
▶ If you are stressed or worried, use your journal to write down your worries and anxieties *before* you go to sleep—then leave them there by set-

ting aside the notebook for tomorrow. This is very effective if you have a busy schedule as well—write down what needs to be done—then leave it there.

▸ Living a sedentary life can affect the quality of sleep you get. Scheduling time to move your body will markedly help you fall asleep and stay asleep.

▸ Take 1 to 4 milligrams of melatonin thirty minutes before sleep. You might want to try the sublingual spray.

▸ Stop drinking caffeine early in the afternoon. Caffeine has a five-hour half-life and can keep you up at night even if you haven't had any for hours.

▸ Allow yourself time to wind down. Don't start new projects in the evening.

▸ If you are having trouble falling asleep, try staring up at the ceiling and counting down from 60: gazing upward stimulates the parasympathetic nervous system, which lowers blood pressure and slows the pace of the breath. Slow, deliberate counting will also help rid your mind of distractions.

▸ Imagine floating on a cloud. What would you see passing by? Guided imagery is a powerful meditation tool that can give you a temporary escape from everyday worries and stresses. Invite all your senses to participate: imagine what you see, hear, and smell in this peaceful place.

▸ Breathe in through your nose and out through your mouth ten times. Focus on your stomach rising and falling and your breath flowing in and out. Now repeat.

START EXERCISING SMART— AND START TODAY!

Exercise burns fat and helps you maintain weight loss; it can also reduce inflammation and the production of free radicals. Start your own exercise program, and within a short time, you will feel so much better that you'll also be a believer in exercise. Remember, it's always a good idea to visit your doctor and get medical clearance before starting an exercise program. This is true for people of all ages.

If you have been living your life as a couch potato, start off slowly. Get in the habit of exercising by walking around the block, going for a bike ride, joining a Zumba class, or taking a swim. Get a guest pass at a local gym to see if you might enjoy using a stationary bike. If you have a Y nearby, and you enjoy the water, ask the staff if they have classes in deep or shallow water aerobics. This is a great way to break into an exercise regime. Water aerobics—low impact or no impact—is easy on your joints. It's also fun. Many Y's and gyms also have less demanding classes in yoga or Pilates, which are good ways to become more accustomed to exercising your body.

Warning: Don't be one of those people who say they can't exercise until they lose weight because they are too embarrassed about how they look. I hear this all the time. This attitude is a recipe for failure. The fact is that everybody feels a little bit exposed and out of place in gym clothes or bathing suits. People are typically so concerned with how they look that they don't really notice anybody else. Start hanging out at the gym, and you'll see what I mean. Get over any sense of being self-conscious and keep focusing on your fat-loss goal.

Just start moving and doing something regularly. It doesn't take long before you will begin feeling more confident about your body. Gradually increase the length of time you spend on the activity and then begin experimenting with other forms of exercise. If you need a push to keep you on track, ask a friend to join you or join a group. If you have a dog, I can guarantee that your pet will be thrilled to join you for longer walks.

If you absolutely prefer exercising alone at home, make a commitment to a definite time schedule and keep it. A personal fitness trainer might also help you get started. Finally, don't put off exercising because you don't have the right equipment. Research some exercise videos that will help you stay focused and that don't require any additional equipment.

HIIT—The Smart Exercise

As you become stronger and more confident about exercise, I'd like you to learn about a smart new form of exercise called high-intensity interval training. HIIT, as it is known, has changed the dynamics of fitness and weight loss.

For years, most of us thought that if we wanted all the fat loss and health benefits of exercise, we had to do it for long periods of time. The longer the cardio or aerobic session, the better. That's what we honestly believed. How times have changed!

We now know there are potential problems with this "the more, the better" approach to exercise, because long bouts of slow and steady aerobic or cardio exercise create low-level systemic inflammation. In fact, these workouts promote oxidative stress, which means more free radicals running around our bodies creating tissue damage and muscle wasting. This type of steady exercise also triggers "pesky"cortisol. Remember, when in excess, cortisol encourages fat storage and the continuation of FATflammation.

If you have found the prospect of long sessions of steady cardio tedious as well as boring, you are going to be much happier with HIIT. Don't let the name scare you off. All HIIT means is that you will be exercising in short intense bursts followed by a period of slowdown and recovery.

The muscles in your body are divided into three categories known as slow twitch, fast twitch, and super fast twitch. When you engage in aerobic exercise like swimming, the slow twitch muscles in your body are the first to contract. As you continue to move, the fast twitch muscles jump in and become part of the action. When you are engaged in a high-intensity exercise like jumping rope or sprinting, your fast twitch muscles are the first to contract. Here's what you need to know: your fast twitch muscles burn more calories and energy faster and can also increase muscle mass more rapidly. HIIT engages all three types of muscle fibers, especially the fast twitch muscles.

Have you ever wondered why so many people (perhaps even you?) spend hours on the treadmill without losing a pound? Tara, one of my clients, was a good example of this. She would walk for miles and also use her elliptical machine for forty minutes at a moderate intensity, and she did it consistently, as many as five times a week. But her weight didn't budge. When she and I began to work together, I introduced her to HIIT and almost immediately, she began to lose weight and her energy soared.

Compared to longer, slower cardio, HIIT increases heart strength and lung power, and you burn more fat and calories than you do with traditional aerobics—and YOU CONTINUE TO DO SO for up to forty-eight hours *after* you exercise. That's right: HIIT continues to help you burn off your weight even after you have stopped exercising. People don't realize that most of the benefits of exercise occur after you are finished. By engaging both your fast twitch and your super fast twitch muscles, you will be burning fat 24/7. Also, the fast twitch muscles you are using release human growth hormone (HGH) by up to 450 percent in the twenty-four hours after you have exercised. HGH is considered the youth hormone because of its ability to keep us leaner, healthier, and more youthful—inside and out. HIIT helps our bodies learn to burn fat after we exercise.

HIIT Benefits
- Burns more fat and calories for up to forty-eight hours after you have finished exercising
- Boosts metabolism
- Superquick workouts
- Keeps and builds muscle mass
- Can be done anywhere
- No equipment needed
- Not boring

If you are a busy person with a million and one things you have to do every day, here's the best thing about HIIT: it takes up much less of your time.

High-Intensity Interval Training— How to Do It

To get a sense of what HIIT is, let's start with a walking exercise. All you have to do is walk as fast as you can for thirty seconds. Then slow down and walk at a moderate speed for ninety seconds. That's it. You exercise intensely for a short period of time (30 seconds) and then you slow it down for a slightly longer period of time (90 seconds). Each of these periods of intense exercise followed by a slowdown is known as an interval. For HIIT, it is usually recommended that you do each of these intervals eight times. If you were to do eight of these intervals, you would be exercising for a total of sixteen minutes. That's all.

There are many variations of HIIT. When you are ready to begin using HIIT for your exercise, remember, if you can only do one interval, do just one. Don't push yourself. You will know when it is time to add another interval. If you are just beginning, take longer rests during the rest phase until you feel comfortable enough to go on. Remember, if you don't have any prior aerobic or strength-training experience or you have been living a sedentary life, begin by walking to build up your fitness level.

You can practice HIIT on any machine or with just about any exercise. You can do it in the pool, on a stationary bike, a treadmill, or an elliptical machine. If you want to do it using machines, I would suggest that you start out working with a fitness professional. Most gyms and Y's have people there to advise you. You can also do it at home employing simple exercises such as push-ups, lunges, chin-ups, or any other exercise you enjoy. There is a great deal of information about HIIT online.

Strength Training

Strength training is also known as weight training or resistance training. Whatever you call it, it builds muscle—AND MUSCLE BURNS FAT. That's all you need to know.

This type of training is just as important for women as it is for men. Women *do not* need to be afraid of becoming muscle-bound because of weight training. Unless they are using drugs or steroids, women don't have high enough testosterone levels to get the huge bulky muscle development you see on men.

It bears repeating that strength training accelerates weight loss, and it doesn't take a lot of time. Two to three times a week of overall strength-training sessions will kick your metabolism into high gear and help you burn fat all day. The combination of HIIT and strength training is superpowerful. Strength training alone has been shown to boost metabolism for twenty-four to forty-eight hours. Strength training has an enormous impact on building the mitochondria—which are the little factories in your cells that burn energy—even while you sleep.

What type of strength training should you do? Start with anything that challenges your muscles. If you've never done any kind of strength training, it's probably wisest to start out in a gym with a trainer or somebody who can show you how to use the appropriate machines.

I have much more in-depth fitness information for you on my website at www.DrLoriShemek.com.

Don't Forget to Stretch

Can you touch your toes? Flexibility is an important component of optimal fitness. When I first became involved with an exercise program, most people were told to stretch before they started. That advice has also changed. We are now told that stretching cold muscles can create problems and that it's wisest to stretch after exercise, when our muscles are all warmed up. One of the great benefits of stretching is that it helps with posture and keeps you looking longer and leaner. To learn how to do it correctly, take a yoga class or get a yoga DVD. Yoga, which incorporates balance along with flexibility, is a great way to become stronger and more confident about your body.

MAINTAIN YOUR DETERMINATION

Staying focused is the biggest challenge for many people trying to lose weight. I would like to tell you about two of my clients. Ken, one of my most memorable clients, consulted me because he was realistically concerned about his health. I have to say that working with Ken was an amazing experience because once he made up his mind to lose his fat, he never lost his focus. When I make home visits to clients, I often do a quick check of the kind of food they are keeping in the kitchen. I visited Ken about a month or so after he started on the diet, and I got to see what was in his refrigerator and pantry. One look, and I recognized the seriousness of his commitment. There was nothing in his kitchen that could tempt him to get off track. Nothing! Ken never wavered. He followed the diet; he took all the recommended supplements; he started exercising; and he kept exercising. He always made sure he had food choices available that were consistent with a FATflammation-free life. When he went to work, he packed his lunch and snacks in a cooler. He bought a fancy water bottle and kept it filled. He took the time to examine his life and note all the things that might distract him or trigger an eating spree. And there were many elements in his life that could have distracted him—high-powered job, family, friends. But he let nothing come between him and his goal to lose weight and get healthy. Ken lost more than two hundred pounds, and he has kept it off.

Delia is another client of mine. She wanted to lose about thirty pounds, and after she went on the diet, she quickly lost about twenty of them in the first five weeks. Then, life with all its distractions got in the way; she lost focus and reverted back to her old habits. When I spoke to Delia, it was apparent that she understood what had happened: she was very aware that her determination had wavered; and she had failed to do the necessary planning and preparing on a regular basis. When she got hungry, she didn't have good anti-inflammatory foods available in her own kitchen, and she had allowed many inflammatory food choices back into her immediate environment. She also became complacent and stopped journaling. Delia told me that her problems started on her birthday. Somebody made her a cake, and she had a piece of it. Then, because she had a piece of cake, she had some ice cream to go with it. That would have okay, if it had stopped there, but it didn't. The day after her birthday, she finished the remains of the cake, which was in her refrigerator. Then, because she figured she had already done the damage,

Delia went on an eating spree of mostly refined carbohydrates that lasted for several weeks. She gained back close to twelve pounds of her original weight before she was able to get herself back on track. Delia was very upset, because more than anything else she wanted her children, particularly her daughters, to have a good role model. Delia was able to stop herself, but she had to go back to the beginning and start all over again. Fortunately Delia was able to recognize the behavior patterns and thought processes that caused her to lose focus.

USE YOUR MIND TO MELT THE FAT

The right mind-set lays the foundation for weight-loss success. If you want to shrink your fat cells, it's essential that you stay positive. Some people feel that their weight gain is beyond their control. They throw their hands up in the air and say, "Forget it, it's not in the cards for me," or they resign themselves to the false notion that "This is my lot in life." Nothing could be further from the truth.

The basis of a healthy mind-set in terms of getting rid of FATflammation is to understand, and fully believe, that you deserve to be at a good and healthy weight. To take that first step on your road to success, you have to place a strong, positive value on who you are and what you deserve. Know that you deserve to feel great about yourself! Acknowledging how incredibly unique and worthwhile you are will take you to where you want to be.

Sometimes, the way we perceive ourselves sets us up for failure. We get stuck in old patterns of thinking. We don't understand that we have the power to make good things happen. Your goal of shrinking your fat cells is important to your happiness. Keep reminding yourself that your goals have great value because YOU have great value. You can make it happen!

Start by introducing more positive thinking into your mind on a daily basis. Doing this is not about being a Pollyanna, nor is it about being in denial. It's just a way of signaling yourself and the universe that you want a positive outcome. Negative thoughts make it very easy to lose focus and give up. Men and women who muster better, more positive thoughts, no matter what the circumstances or situation, tend to be more successful in all their endeavors.

Visualizations to Improve Your Mind-Set

I always like to remind clients about the power of visualization. Visualization techniques are used by top-level athletes as a way of helping them excel in their given sports. Athletes from the Soviet Union and Germany were at the forefront of this practice, and many say it was one of the reasons why these countries dominated at many world-class events for years, before the rest of the world caught on. Visualization works because the mind can't differentiate between something that is real and something that is imagined. Research shows that simply by thinking about your goal as if the goal had already been accomplished you strengthen neuronal pathways in the brain. If you're not sure what visualization actually is, just stop for a minute and think about a fond memory. Let the memory settle into your head. Look at everything that is taking place in your memory. That's visualization.

Now visualize something you want for yourself in the future. View your goal (any goal you have) as a movie in which you are playing the starring role. Just close your eyes and, with as much detail as possible, create a scene. Bring your senses into play. What do you see? What do you hear? Is it a beautiful spring day? Can you smell the flowers? When you add your senses to your visualization, you are making it that much more real.

Each day, take a few minutes to visualize or imagine, in your mind, what a successful day would be for you. Visualize your weight-loss goals as though you have already been successful in making them happen. In your mind's eye, see yourself wearing the clothes you want to be wearing. Use the sense of touch and imagine what the fabric feels like. See yourself playing a sport you want to play; see yourself walking down the street and pausing to look in a store window, happy at the sight of the image reflected back at you. See yourself looking and feeling the way you want to look and feel. Do this each day when you first wake up and then again before you fall asleep. Embed in your mind the idea and image of yourself as a thin, vibrant, happy, and healthy person.

CHAPTER 17

DON'T FORGET ABOUT SUPPLEMENTS

▶ Supplements are an essential part of the FATflammation-Free Diet Program. I firmly believe supplements will help you be more successful in reaching your weight-loss goals. Consistency in remembering to take your supplements is key.

These are the supplements I suggest to my clients. Before taking any supplement, it's always a good idea to discuss it with your doctor or health care professional. If you are under medical supervision for any ongoing medical conditions, it's essential that you do this. Never take more than the recommended dose. Do not, for example, assume that because one green tea capsule might help you lose weight, you should be doubling or tripling the amount to lose even more weight. Some people have become ill doing this. Remember that supplements are important tools for healing, and they can be very powerful. Also please remember to take your supplements with food. The only exception to this is glucomannan, which is a fiber.

MULTIVITAMIN AND MINERAL (WITHOUT IRON)
Dosage Recommendation: 1 daily

Few of us are getting all the vitamins we need. A good multivitamin gives us extra protection.

OMEGA-3 FISH OIL (PURIFIED)
Dosage Recommendation: 4,000 mg daily

Fish oil is a source of omega-3 fatty acids. It reduces inflammation, decreases appetite, increases insulin sensitivity, balances blood sugar, and helps build muscle. Fish oil is critical for weight-loss success and is one of the most effective tools we have to help us break the weight/inflammation cycle.

Vegetarians and vegans can use the following omega-3 supplement.

ALGAE-DERIVED DHA OMEGA-3 SUPPLEMENT
Dosage Recommendation: 350 mg (as directed) DHA, 50 mg EPA daily

DHA is an essential (meaning the only way to get this fatty acid is from your diet) omega-3 fat, which is critical for weight loss. By increasing your omega-3 fat intake via algae (which is how fish get theirs), you are helping to maintain a healthy omega-3/omega-6 balance. If you want to reverse FATflammation, this is absolutely necessary.

ASTAXANTHIN
Dosage Recommendation: 4 mg daily

Astaxanthin, a carotenoid, is a powerful anti-inflammatory found in vegetables, salmon, algae, and other marine life. Inflamed fat cells have a reduction in fat-burning hormones. Astaxanthin increases your body's sensitivity to insulin.

B VITAMIN COMPLEX
Dosage Recommendation: 100 mg daily

B complex can help make your metabolism become more efficient. These nutrients help metabolize fat, protein, and carbohydrates. The B vitamins B_6, folate, and B_{12} help reduce inflammation. It is important to take a B complex as opposed to taking individual B vitamins separately. B vitamins act together synergistically. Taking one alone can create a deficiency of another. B vitamins help to stop cravings when taken in conjunction with chromium picolinate.

VITAMIN C

Dosage Recommendation: 2,000 mg daily

Vitamin C is an antioxidant that can help reduce inflammation in the body. It is also required for the metabolism of fatty tissue. Without sufficient vitamin C, your body is unable to use stored fat. A low vitamin C level is linked with increased weight and a higher waist measurement.

VITAMIN D₃

Dosage Recommendation: 3,000–4,000 IUs daily

Have your blood tested before you start taking a vitamin D₃ supplement so that you have a baseline—retest in six months to achieve optimal level. There is a link between weight gain, insulin resistance, and vitamin D (a pro-hormone) deficiency. When the brain senses low vitamin D levels, it triggers the release of hunger hormones encouraging overeating. Vitamin D is effective for all-over fat reduction but particularly belly fat. Several studies also show that insufficient levels of vitamin D can put you at risk for a variety wide variety of health issues, including arthritis, heart disease, and cancer. A recent study also showed that women with the highest levels of vitamin D had a much higher rate of survival from breast cancer than those with lower levels.

ACETYL L-CARNITINE

Dosage Recommendation: 500 mg daily

Acetyl L-carnitine is an antioxidant that helps your body absorb and metabolize dietary fats. Acetyl L-carnitine can improve energy and also helps boost the level of the weight-loss hormone adiponectin.

R-LIPOIC ACID

Dosage Recommendation: 400 mg daily

R-lipoic acid helps weight loss by triggering mechanisms that stop the storage of fat and has the ability to balance blood sugar. *Bonus:* R-lipoic acid regenerates vitamins E and C—both necessary for reducing inflammation.

CHROMIUM PICOLINATE
Dosage Recommendation: 400 mcg daily

This mineral packs a powerful weight-loss punch. It helps stop sugar and carbohydrate cravings by balancing the blood sugar. Studies have found that chromium picolinate can help to decrease body fat and increase lean muscle mass while balancing blood sugar. This is key to reducing hunger, cravings, and inflammation.

GREEN TEA EXTRACT
Dosage Recommendation: 400 mg daily

One of the more powerful compounds in green tea is the antioxidant epigallocatechin gallate (EGCG), which has been shown to increase metabolism and burn fat for energy.

MAGNESIUM
Dosage Recommendation: 400 mg daily

Magnesium is required for every process in the human body and is powerful in reducing inflammation and oxidative stress. It is an important key in helping the body utilize proteins, carbohydrates, and fats. Magnesium plays an important role in balancing blood sugar.

MILK THISTLE
Dosage Recommendation: 150 mg daily

Milk thistle supports liver health. Many people who are overweight also have fatty liver. Milk thistle can help your liver cells regenerate and help you create a healthy new liver (remember, it's your number one fat-burning organ).

N-ACETYL CYSTEINE (NAC)
Dosage Recommendation: 500 mg daily

N-acetyl cysteine (NAC) is an amino acid and powerful antioxidant that decreases insulin's effect at the fat cell and helps aid weight loss by reducing fat storage. It helps your liver function!

COENZYME Q10 (COQ10)
Dosage Recommendation: 150 mg daily

CoQ10 is essential for the breakdown of fat. This powerful antioxidant can help protect against oxidative damage from free radicals. A deficiency of CoQ10 may result in less energy and a slower metabolism. CoQ10 decreases naturally with age.

CURCUMIN
Dosage Recommendation: 400 mg daily

Curcumin is a powerful anti-inflammatory and has the ability to stop the growth of fat tissue leading to weight loss and the prevention of obesity.

RESVERATROL
Dosage Recommendation: 250 mg daily

Resveratrol is a powerful antioxidant that can help protect against inflammation and balance blood sugar.

PROBIOTICS
Dosage Recommendation: One capsule, 15 Billion CFUs (colony-forming units), daily

Probiotics can help reduce belly fat and all-over weight. Beneficial bacteria help manage cortisol and maintain healthy insulin levels. Probiotics help maintain a healthy gut by fighting inflammation in the digestive tract.

GLUCOMANNAN FIBER SUPPLEMENT
(FOLLOW PRODUCT INSTRUCTIONS)

Dosage Recommendation: 2.5 g (30 minutes before each meal)

Glucomannan is a fiber supplement that helps stabilize blood sugar, supports healthy insulin function, promotes a sense of fullness, and can help control food cravings. The brand I take is PGX. Be certain to drink all the recommended water.

Allowed Foods and Recipes

FATFLAMMATION-FREE
COMPLETE FOODS LIST

FAT-BURNING PROTEINS

(One serving equals the size and thickness of your hand including fingers.)

Eggs

Free range

Organic

Regular eggs

Poultry—When possible, choose natural or organic

Canned chicken

Chicken (all cuts, skinless)

Duck breast

Ground chicken (drained of fat)

Ground turkey (drained of fat)

Turkey breast or thighs (skinless)

Meat—When possible, choose natural, grass-fed, and/or buy organic

Beef tenderloin

Buffalo/bison

Flank steak

Game meats

Lean ground beef

Lean lamb

Pork tenderloin

Pot roast

Prime rib

Round steak

Sirloin steak

Skirt steak

Veal chop or roast

Lean Naturally Processed Meats—*Ensure a minimum of 4 grams of protein per fat gram*

Canadian bacon	Roast beef slices
Chicken sausage	Turkey bacon
Chicken slices	Turkey sausage
Lean bacon (nitrate/nitrite free)	Turkey slices

Seafood—*When possible, choose wild caught*

Anchovies	Perch
Bass	Pollack
Black sea bass	Prawns
Catfish	Red snapper
Chilean sea bass	Salmon—fresh and canned
Clams	(chinook, chum, coho, pink,
Cod	naturally farmed, pink,
Crab	sockeye)
Crawfish	Sardines (water-packed)
Flounder/sole	Scallops
Grouper	Shark
Haddock	Shrimp
Halibut	Sole
Herring	Squid
Lobster	Swordfish
Monkfish	Trout
Mussels	Tuna (fresh and canned)
Oysters	White fish

FRUITS

(One serving = size of your fist)

Apple	**Lemon**
Blackberries	**Lime**
Blueberries	**Loganberries**
Boysenberries	**Pear**
Cherries (tart, not sweet)	**Raspberries**
Gooseberries	**Rhubarb**
Grapefruit	**Strawberries**
Kiwi	

Juice

Freshly juiced green veggies	**Low-sodium tomato**
Low-sodium veggie juice	

FIGHTING FATFLAMMATION WITH VEGETABLES

(Unlimited servings unless otherwise specified)

Alfalfa sprouts	**Broccolini**
Artichokes	**Brussels sprouts**
Arugula	**Burdock**
Asparagus	**Cabbage**
Avocados (one serving =	**Carrots (raw and in moderation)**
½ avocado)	**Cassava**
Bamboo shoots	**Cauliflower**
Bell peppers (green, red,	**Celery**
orange, yellow, purple)	**Collard greens**
Bok choy	**Cucumber**
Broccoli	**Daikon**

Dandelion greens
Eggplant
Endive
Fennel
Green onions
Jicama
Kale
Kohlrabi
Leek
Lettuce
Mushrooms (all varieties)
Mustard greens
Okra
Onion
Parsnips

Pickles
Radicchio
Radishes
Sprouts (all varieties)
Sauerkraut
Seaweed (all varieties)
Spinach
Summer squash
Swiss chard
Tomatoes
Tomatillas
Turnip greens
Watercress
Zucchini

STARCHY CARBS

Pumpkin
Rutabaga
Spaghetti squash
Squash (acorn, butternut, winter)

Sweet potatoes (one serving =
    ½ fist)
Turnip
Yams (one serving = ½ fist)

LEGUMES

(One serving = one fist)

Adzuki beans
Bean sprouts
Black beans
Black-eyed peas

Black soy beans
Butter beans
Cannellini beans
Cow peas

Edamame

Fava beans

Garbanzo beans (chickpea)

Green beans

Kidney beans

Lentils

Lentil sprouts

Lima beans

Mung beans

Navy beans

Peas

Red beans

Refried beans (without hydrogenated trans fat)

Split peas

Soybeans

White beans

DAIRY SELECTIONS

Almond milk (unsweetened)

Almond or rice-based cheeses (vegetarian)

Butter (preferably organic, grass-fed)

Buttermilk

Cheese (low fat)

Coconut butter

Coconut milk (unsweetened)

Cottage cheese (low fat, plain)

Cream cheese (low fat)

Cream cheese substitute (low fat)

Goat cheese

Grass-fed milk

Greek yogurt (2% plain)

Hard cheeses

Hemp milk (unsweetened)

Kefir (low fat, plain)

Organic milk (2%)

Parmesan cheese

Provolone cheese

Ricotta (part-skim)

Sour cream (nonfat, low fat)

String cheese

Swiss cheese

Yogurt (2%, plain)

PROTEIN SUPPLEMENTS

Whey protein powder

Vegan powdered pea-rice protein

GRAINS (IN MODERATION)

Amaranth

Black rice

Brown rice

Buckwheat

Cracked wheat

Farro

Hull-less barley

Kamut (contains gluten)

Kasha

Millet

Quinoa

Red rice

Rye

Spelt (contains gluten)

Sprouted whole grains

*Steel-cut oats (oats are gluten free but may be contaminated with wheat during processing)

Teff

Wheat berries (contains gluten)

Whole wheat

Wild pecan rice

Wild rice

FAT-BURNING FATS

All nuts and seeds oils

Almond oil

Avocado oil

Coconut oil

Flax oil

Ghee (clarified butter; *can be used in week 1—contains no dairy)

Macadamia nut oil (cold-pressed)

Olive oil

Organic butter

FLOURS

Almond (gluten free, best for baking)

Amaranth (gluten free)

Arrowroot (gluten free, thickener)

Barley

Brown rice (gluten free)

Chickpea (gluten free)

Coconut (gluten free, best for baking)

Hazelnut (gluten free, best for baking)

Millet (gluten free)

Pecan (gluten free, best for baking)

Quinoa (gluten free)

Teff

Whole wheat

FAT-RELEASING CONDIMENTS AND SEASONINGS

(Serving size = unlimited amounts unless otherwise specified)

All fresh or dried spices

Basil

Bay leaves

Cinnamon

Cumin

Garlic

Horseradish

Hot sauce

Ketchup (without sugar, or HFCS use in moderation)

Lemon juice

Mustard (all varieties, especially hot mustard)

Peppers and peppercorns (hot chile, black, white, pink, green)

Pickles

Salsa

Turmeric

Vinegar

Wasabi powder

FAT-BURNING DIPS

(Serving size = ½ fist)

Black bean

Guacamole

Hummus

Lentil

NUTS

Almonds	Macadamia nuts	Pistachios
Brazil nuts	Peanuts	Walnuts
Cashews	Pecan	
Hazelnuts	Pine nuts	

SEEDS

Chia	Poppy	Sesame
Flax (ground only)	Pumpkin	Sunflower
Hemp		

NUT BUTTERS

Almond	Macadamia	Pistachio
Cashew	Peanut	Walnut
Hazelnut	Pecan	

BEVERAGES

All herbal teas (Rooiboos, green tea, dandelion root)	Kombucha tea drink
Black tea	Stevia-sweetened sodas
Green tea	White tea

SWEETENERS

Just Like Sugar	Stevia
Swerve	Xylitol
Pure Monk Fruit Sweetener	Yacon syrup

MISCELLANEOUS ACCEPTABLE LOW-CARB CHOICES

Low-carb bread made with almond/coconut flour

Low-carb coconut wraps

Low-carb English muffins

Low-carb tortillas

Morningstar Farms Sausage Patties (low-carb vegetarian)

Shirataki noodles (noodles with virtually no carb)

SNACKS

See page 269 for more snack ideas.

Beef, turkey, or salmon jerky

Olives

Pickles

Roasted chickpeas or garbanzo beans

Thin crisp breads such as Rye-Vita

CULTURED FOODS

Dark chocolate (over 70% cacao)

Kefir

Kimchi

Natto

Pickled ginger

Pickles

Sauerkraut

Vegetables

Yogurt

FATFLAMMATION-FREE
DIET PROGRAM RECIPES

Scrambled Eggs with Avocado, Sun-Dried Tomatoes, and Mushrooms

    1 tablespoon butter or olive oil
    ½ portobello mushroom, diced
    2 whole medium-size eggs
    1 tablespoon chopped sun-dried tomatoes
    ¼ diced small avocado
    Salt and pepper to taste

Heat 1 tablespoon butter or olive oil over medium heat. Put the chopped tomato and mushrooms in the hot skillet; season with salt and pepper. Whisk the eggs with avocado and add to the skillet. When the eggs have begun to set at the edges, use spatula or wooden spoon to scrape the eggs from the edge of the pan to the center. Cook until the eggs are set but still slightly moist, about 5 minutes.

Serves 1

Texas Skillet Turkey Dinner

1 pound ground turkey

½ cup chopped onion

3 garlic cloves, minced

1 (14-ounce) can diced tomatoes, undrained

1 (15-ounce) can red kidney beans, drained

1 (4-ounce) can chopped green chili peppers

3 tablespoons chopped bell peppers, any color

1½ teaspoons chili powder

1½ teaspoons ground cumin

½ teaspoon salt

½ cup water

In a nonstick skillet, cook ground turkey, onion, and garlic until meat is browned and vegetables are tender. Stir in the undrained tomatoes, beans, green chili peppers, bell peppers, chili powder, cumin, salt, and water. Cover and bring to a simmer for 20 minutes.

Serves 4

Avocado Arugula Salad with Blueberries

2 cups arugula

¼ diced avocado

¼ cup blueberries

2 tablespoons diced red onion

1 tablespoon macadamia nut oil

1 tablespoon balsamic vinegar, vinegar, or lemon juice

Chop and mix all vegetables. Add blueberries. Drizzle macadamia nut oil and balsamic vinegar over salad. Mix gently.

Serves 1

Lori's Spicy Chai Smoothie

> 1 scoop vanilla whey protein powder
> (or pea-rice protein powder)
> ½ cup almond milk
> ½ cup chilled brewed chai tea
> 1 tablespoon coconut oil
> 1 cup ice cubes
> ½ teaspoon cinnamon

Combine all ingredients in blender. Blend until smooth.

Serves 1

Tuna-Pistachio Stuffed Tomatoes

> 2 large tomatoes
> 6 ounces tuna packed in water, drain well
> 1 tablespoon capers (optional)
> 1 tablespoon chopped onion
> 2 tablespoons chopped pistachios
> 2 tablespoons chopped parsley
> 1 tablespoon lemon juice
> 1 tablespoon macadamia nut oil
> Salt and pepper to taste

Slice the top off each tomato. Scoop out the inside of the tomato. Keep only the tomato flesh and discard the seeds. In a medium bowl, combine that remaining tomato flesh with the tuna, onion, pistachio, capers, parsley, lemon juice, macadamia nut oil, salt, and pepper. Divide the mixture and stuff each tomato. Serve immediately or refrigerate.

Serves 2

Spinach and Bean Sauté

1 15-ounce can cannellini or white beans, rinsed and drained
1 tablespoon macadamia nut oil
½ diced onion
2 small garlic cloves, chopped
2 cups spinach leaves
¼ cup low-sodium chicken broth (optional)
Salt and pepper to taste

Add macadamia nut oil to pan and sauté onion and garlic until soft. Add in beans to warm through. Add spinach and cook until wilted. Salt and pepper to taste. Use the chicken broth to loosen the dish up if necessary.

Serves 2

Turkey Hummus BLT Wrap

2 slices cooked turkey bacon
3 ounces cooked turkey breast (sliced or diced)
2 tablespoons hummus
Sliced tomato
Lettuce
Coconut wrap (or substitute lettuce as a wrap)

Spread hummus on the coconut wrap. Place the bacon evenly on wrap and top the wrap with turkey, tomato, and lettuce. Roll tightly

Serves 1

3-Bean Beef Chili

2 tablespoons olive oil
1½ pounds lean ground beef or buffalo

   1 15-ounce can red kidney beans, rinsed and drained

   1 15-ounce can black beans, rinsed and drained

   1 15-ounce can great northern beans, rinsed and drained

   1 28-ounce can no-salt diced tomatoes

   2 cups water or low-sodium chicken broth

   1 onion, diced

   3 garlic cloves, minced

   ¼ cup chili powder

   ½ tablespoon oregano

   ½ tablespoon cumin

In a medium pot, brown beef, onion, and garlic in oil until onion has softened. Add in the beans, tomatoes, water or chicken broth, chili powder, oregano, and cumin. Bring to a boil. Reduce heat to low/medium, cover, and simmer 30 to 45 minutes until thickened. (Can be frozen and used for another meal.)

   Serves 6

Ground Turkey Stuffed Peppers

   1 tablespoon olive oil

   1 pound ground turkey breast

   1 small onion, finely chopped

   1 15-ounce can of black beans, rinsed and drained

   1 8-ounce can of tomato sauce

   1 28-ounce can of diced Italian-style tomatoes

   Salt and pepper

   4 medium-size green peppers

Brown turkey and onion over medium heat. Once turkey is browned, stir in black beans, tomato sauce, salt and pepper. Bring to a boil then reduce heat to a simmer. Cover and cook for 15 minutes. While the turkey mixture is cooking, preheat the oven to 350°F. Next, remove stem end from peppers and remove seeds and membrane from the inside of pepper. Evenly stuff each pepper with turkey mixture. Arrange in shallow baking dish. Pour 28-ounce canned tomatoes over all four peppers. Bake at 350°F for 40 minutes.

Serves 4

Berry Coconut Yogurt Smoothie

   4 ounces of plain, unsweetened cultured coconut yogurt (plain 2% Greek yogurt may be substituted)

   ½ scoop of whey protein

   ½ cup of unsweetened almond milk or any other type of nondairy milk

   1 cup of frozen berries

   1 tablespoon coconut oil

   1 to 2 drops of liquid stevia (optional: have unsweetened or choose another allowed sweetener from list on page 228)

Combine all ingredients in blender. Blend until smooth.

Serves 1

Chicken Marinara

   4 boneless skinless chicken breasts

   1 tablespoon macadamia nut oil

   3 garlic cloves, crushed

   1 cup sliced mushrooms (any variety)

   ¼ cup of chopped black or green olives

   ½ teaspoon dried basil

   1 24-ounce jar of marinara sauce (no added sugar)

Heat macadamia nut oil until hot. Add chicken breasts and cook until browned on each side. Remove from pan and set aside. Add garlic, mushrooms, olives, and basil to the pan. Sauté until mushrooms are tender. Add in browned chicken and marinara sauce. Simmer for 15 minutes or until heated through.

Serves 4

Coconut Chocolate Milk Smoothie

- 1 scoop chocolate whey protein
- 1 handful of spinach or kale
- 1 tablespoon cocoa powder (optional)
- 2 cups unsweetened coconut milk
- 4 ice cubes
- Dash cinnamon
- Dash almond extract
- 1 to 2 drops of liquid stevia (optional: have unsweetened or choose another allowed sweetener from list on page 228)

Combine all ingredients in blender. Blend until smooth.

Serves 2

Lentil and Turkey Sausage Soup

- 2 tablespoons olive oil
- 12 ounces medium sliced turkey sausage (any variety of turkey sausage)
- 1 small onion, chopped
- 1 rib of celery, diced
- 1 clove garlic, minced
- 4 cups low-sodium chicken broth

2 15-ounce cans lentils, rinsed and drained

1 14-ounce can diced tomatoes

1 bay leaf

Salt and pepper

Heat oil in large saucepan. Add sausage and cook over medium heat until browned on each side. Add onion and celery and cook until softened. Add garlic and sauté for 1 minute. Add chicken broth, lentils, tomatoes, and bay leaf. Salt and pepper to taste. Bring to a boil. Reduce heat, cover, and simmer for 45 minutes. (Can be frozen for another meal)

Serves 4

WEEK TWO RECIPES

Spinach, Feta Cheese, and Mushroom Omelet

2 medium-size eggs

1 cup fresh spinach

¼ cup sliced mushrooms

1 teaspoon macadamia nut oil

1 tablespoon feta cheese

Pepper

Whisk two eggs. Heat oil in a small skillet over medium heat. Add spinach and mushrooms, sauté until spinach is wilted and mushrooms are heated through. Add eggs. Cook until eggs are firm. Crumble feta cheese over top of omelet, fold in half.

Serves 1

Chicken Nuggets

2 tablespoons extra-virgin olive oil

¾ pound skinless boneless chicken breasts

¾ cup of almond flour

1 tablespoon poultry seasoning

1 teaspoon dried parsley

1 teaspoon garlic powder

1 teaspoon paprika

Salt and pepper

Preheat oven to 400°F. Coat baking sheet with oil. Cut chicken into 1-inch nugget pieces and set aside. In a large mixing bowl, combine almond flour and all seasonings. Coat all surfaces of chicken pieces in mixture. Lay chicken pieces on baking pan and bake for 10 minutes or until slightly browned. Serve.

Serves 2

Almond-Crusted Cod

2 tablespoons macadamia nut oil, divided

1½ pounds of cod cut into four sections

¾ cup coarsely ground almonds

¼ cup chopped parsley

2 teaspoons Italian seasoning

Salt and pepper to taste

1 whole medium-size egg and 3 egg whites

4 lemon wedges for garnish

Preheat oven to 420°F. Coat baking sheet with 1 tablespoon of oil. Combine almonds, parsley, Italian seasoning, salt, and pepper until well mixed. Set aside. Whisk together the whole egg with the egg whites. Coat each section of fish with egg wash and then coat fish with ground almond mixture. Place fish pieces on baking sheet and drizzle with 1 tablespoon of oil. Cook for 15 minutes or until fish flakes easily with a fork. Serve with lemon wedges.

Serves 4

Kale and Mashed Avocado Salad

1 bunch kale (any variety), with ribs removed and torn into
   bite-size pieces
1 very ripened avocado, mashed
Juice of ½ lemon
¼ teaspoon minced garlic

Mix kale and avocado until kale leaves are completely coated. Add in lemon juice and garlic and mix well.

Serves 2–3

Julie's Greek Chicken Soup with Brown Rice

1 chicken breast bone-in, skin removed
1 quart (32 ounces) low-sodium chicken broth
¼ cup brown rice
2 cups fresh spinach, packed tightly
1 whole medium-size egg
½ cup lemon juice
Salt and pepper to taste

Bring chicken broth to a medium boil. Add chicken and brown rice. Reduce to a low simmer. Cover and cook for 30 minutes until chicken and rice are done. Remove chicken, discard bone, and dice chicken into small pieces. Add diced chicken and spinach to soup. Simmer until spinach is cooked (approximately 1 to 2 minutes). Whisk one egg and drizzle into soup, stirring. Add lemon juice; and salt and pepper.

Serves 2–4

Hot Garlic Shrimp

1 tablespoon olive oil
1 pound large shrimp
2 garlic cloves, finely minced
¼ teaspoon crushed red pepper
Juice of ½ lemon
1 tablespoon parsley
Salt and pepper to taste

Heat olive oil in a large skillet over medium heat. Add garlic and red pepper flakes. Cook for a minute. Add shrimp and sauté until shrimp is pink and tender. Add lemon juice and parsley; season with salt and pepper. Warm through.

Serves 4

Lori's Luscious Smoothie

1 scoop whey protein powder (chocolate/vanilla)
Handful fresh blueberries
¼ avocado
2 tablespoons ground flax seeds
½ teaspoon cinnamon
8 ounces no-sugar coconut milk

Combine all ingredients in blender. Blend until smooth.

Serves 1

Open-Face Tuna Sandwich Melt

1 can or packet of tuna in water, drained

2 tablespoons onion, finely chopped

2 tablespoons celery, chopped

1 tablespoon black olives, chopped

½ tablespoon extra-virgin olive oil

1 tablespoon parsley, chopped

Salt and pepper

3 tablespoons reduced-fat shredded cheese of choice

½ gluten-free sprouted English muffin

In a medium bowl combine tuna, onion, celery, olives, parsley, olive oil, and salt and pepper to taste. Mix ingredients well. Mound tuna mix onto English muffin and sprinkle with shredded cheese. Place under broiler and heat until cheese is melted.

Serves 1

Bean Soup with Smoked Turkey Sausage

2 tablespoons extra-virgin olive oil

1 pound smoked turkey sausage, sliced into ½-inch pieces

1 onion, chopped

3 garlic cloves, finely minced

1 14-ounce can diced tomatoes, not drained

10 ounces fresh spinach

1 bay leaf

2 15-ounce cans of cannellini or any white beans, rinsed and drained

4 cups (32-ounce) low-sodium chicken broth

Salt and pepper to taste

In a large pot over medium heat, heat olive oil. Add smoked sausage and sauté for 5 minutes or until browned. Add onion and garlic, and cook until softened. Add tomatoes, beans, bay leaf, chicken broth, and season with salt and pepper. Add in spinach during last 10 minutes of cooking. Reduce heat and simmer for 30 minutes. (Make ahead for lunch.)

Serves 4

Salmon Burger on a Bed of Mixed Baby Greens

½ cup chopped onion

¼ cup chopped parsley

12 ounces canned salmon, drained

1 whole medium-size egg and 2 egg whites whisked together well

Salt and pepper

1 tablespoon coconut oil

½ cup mixed baby greens tossed with ½ tablespoon olive oil

½ lemon

In a medium bowl combine onion, parsley, salmon, and whisked eggs; salt and pepper to taste. Mix well. Form 2 patties. Heat coconut oil on medium-high heat. Add salmon patties to pan. Cook until browned on each side. Serve over mixed baby greens. Drizzle with lemon juice to taste.

Serves 2

Shrimp and Veggie Stir-Fry

1 tablespoon sesame or coconut oil

6 ounces shrimp

1 teaspoon finely minced garlic

4 ounces mushrooms

½ cup of halved cherry tomatoes

2 cups bok choy or spinach

½ cup cooked brown rice

Add oil to a hot medium skillet or wok. Add shrimp and garlic. Cook shrimp until pink. Add mushrooms, tomatoes, bok choy or spinach, and sauté until veggies are slightly softened yet bright in color. Serve over hot brown rice.

Serves 1

"Pasta" and Turkey Marinara Sauce

> 1 spaghetti squash
> 1 tablespoon coconut oil
> 1 pound ground turkey
> 2 cloves garlic, chopped
> 1 24-ounce jar marinara sauce (no sugar added)
> ⅛ teaspoon hot red pepper flakes (optional) or ground black pepper

Cut spaghetti squash in half lengthwise, and scoop out seeds and membranes. Bake squash at 425°F for 30 to 40 minutes. When done, loosen the squash with a fork, remove, and set aside. In a large heated skillet, add 1 tablespoon coconut oil. Add turkey and garlic. Brown turkey. Add in marinara sauce. Heat through and serve over spaghetti squash "noodles."

Serves 4

Turkey Burger Avocado Wrap

> 4 ounces ground turkey breast
> 1 teaspoon macadamia nut oil
> 1 teaspoon finely diced red onion
> 1 tablespoon chopped parsley
> ½ teaspoon garlic powder
> Salt and pepper to taste
> 1 low-carb gluten-free wrap of choice

¼ avocado, sliced

Salsa to taste

In a large mixing bowl, combine turkey, red onion, parsley, garlic powder, and salt and pepper. Shape into burger patty. Heat small skillet with macadamia nut oil on medium-heat. When pan is hot, add turkey burger. Cook until done. Add burger to wrap. Top burger with avocado and salsa.

Serves 1

Prosciutto-Wrapped Cod

4 4-ounce cod fillets

3 ounces thinly sliced prosciutto

1 tablespoon olive oil

Wrap each filet with 1 to 2 slices of prosciutto. In a medium skillet, heat olive oil over medium heat. Once hot, add wrapped cod filets to pan and cook until prosciutto is crispy and fish is cooked through.

Serves 4

Protein Pancakes

¼ cup whole oats

½ cup low-fat cottage cheese

2 whole medium-size eggs

1 teaspoon coconut oil

Yacon syrup (optional)

Blend oats, cottage cheese, and eggs in blender until smooth. Heat coconut oil in skillet over medium heat. Pour ¼ cup of batter for each pancake. When pancake starts to bubble turn pancake over. Serve hot with yacon syrup.

Serves 1–2

Berry Yogurt Parfait

  4 ounces plain or coconut yogurt
  1 teaspoon ground flax seeds or chia seeds
  5 strawberries, (fresh or unsweetened frozen) sliced
  ¼ cup blueberries (fresh or unsweetened frozen)

Add seeds to yogurt. Mix well. Spoon some of the yogurt mixture into a clear glass and place a layer of strawberries on top of yogurt. Add a layer of blueberries. Add more yogurt and repeat the process.

  Serves 1

Crunchy Mozzarella Salmon Melt

  4 ounces water-packed salmon, drained
  1 tablespoon crushed pecans
  1 slice sprouted gluten-free whole-grain bread
  3 tablespoons shredded mozzarella cheese
  Salt and pepper to taste

In a small mixing bowl, blend salmon, pecans, and salt and pepper. Place salmon mixture on top of gluten-free bread. Sprinkle cheese over top. Broil until heated through and cheese melts.

  Serves 1

Broiled Sirloin Steak

  4- to 6-ounce grass-fed sirloin steak
  2 garlic cloves
  Salt and pepper to taste

Smash garlic cloves on a cutting board with the side of a knife to make a paste. Rub garlic paste on both sides of steak. Season with salt and pepper. Broil steak 4 minutes on each side or until desired doneness.

Serves 1

WEEK THREE RECIPES

Parmesan-Crusted Zucchini Medallions

4 medium zucchini, sliced into ¼-inch rounds
1 tablespoon extra-virgin olive oil
½ cup of grated parmesan cheese
¼ teaspoon dried rosemary
⅛ teaspoon ground pepper

Heat oven to 425°F. In a medium-size bowl, toss zucchini with oil. Mix together parmesan cheese, rosemary, and pepper. Firmly press the cheese mixture onto zucchini medallions. Place zucchini on baking sheet and cook for 20 minutes or until browned and crisp.

Serves 4

Baby Arugula, Avocado, and Tomato Salad

3 cups baby arugula lettuce
1 avocado, diced
¾ cup cherry tomatoes, halved
⅛ cup pine nuts
1 teaspoon finely minced garlic
1 teaspoon coarse mustard

3 tablespoons extra-virgin olive oil
Juice of 1 lemon
Ground pepper to taste

In a large bowl, whisk olive oil, garlic, mustard, and lemon juice. Add in arugula, avocado, tomatoes, pine nuts, and pepper. Toss well to coat all leaves.

Serves 4

Deviled Hummus Eggs

1 medium-size hard-boiled egg
1 tablespoon hummus
Salt and pepper to taste
Paprika

Cut egg in half length-wise. Scoop out yolk and place in small bowl. Add in hummus and salt and pepper. Mix well until smooth. Spoon filling into egg white halves, filling each evenly. Sprinkle with paprika.

Serves 1

Chicken Salad in Pita Pocket

8 ounces of shredded chicken
¼ cup sliced almonds
⅓ cup diced apple
½ cup 2% plain Greek yogurt
¼ teaspoon curry powder
Pepper to taste
3 sprouted-wheat pita pockets

Add chicken to a large bowl. Add almonds, apples, yogurt, curry powder, and pepper. Mix well until all ingredients are coated. Divide and fill pita pockets with chicken salad.

Serves 3

Penne Pasta with Shrimp and Sausage

> 16 ounces brown rice penne pasta
> 3 tablespoons olive oil
> ½ cup of red onion, chopped
> 2 tablespoons chopped garlic
> 1 28-ounce can crushed tomatoes
> ½ pound turkey sausage (diced)
> ½ teaspoon dried oregano
> ½ teaspoon thyme
> ½ teaspoon chili flakes
> Salt and pepper
> 1½ pounds medium shrimp (cleaned and deveined)

Bring a large pot of water to a boil. Add penne pasta and cook for approximately 10 minutes or until al dente. Drain pasta and set aside. Heat the oil in a large skillet over medium heat. Add sausage, onion, oregano, thyme, chili flakes, garlic, salt, and pepper. Cook until sausage is browned and herbs are aromatic. Add crushed tomatoes and simmer for 10 minutes. Add shrimp and simmer until done (about 4 minutes). Ladle sauce onto pasta and serve hot.

Serves 8

Salad Nicoise

> 1 head of Boston or butter lettuce, torn into pieces
> 1 4-ounce packet or can of water-packed tuna, drained

1 ripe tomato, quartered

2 hard-boiled medium-size eggs, quartered

½ cup of whole, pitted black olives

4 to 6 anchovy fillets

1 teaspoon Dijon mustard

2 tablespoons lemon juice

3 tablespoons extra-virgin olive oil

Arrange lettuce on a serving dish and top with tuna, eggs, tomatoes, olives, and anchovies. *For the vinaigrette:* Whisk mustard and lemon juice together well. Slowly whisk in the olive oil. Pour vinaigrette over salad and serve.

Serves 2–3

Walnut Pesto Cod

1 tablespoon extra-virgin olive oil

1 pound cod, divided into four pieces

4 tablespoons store-bought walnut pesto

Salt and pepper to taste

Heat oven to 375°F. Coat medium-size baking dish with olive oil. Sprinkle salt and pepper on cod. Bake fish for 15 minutes or until fish flakes easily with fork. Spoon 1 tablespoon pesto over each piece of cod. Serve hot.

Serves 4

Berry Ginger Smoothie

1 cup 2% plain Greek yogurt

1 tablespoon coconut oil

1 cup almond milk

½-inch piece of ginger root, peeled

2 handfuls of spinach

½ cup frozen (or fresh) blackberries or other berries of choice

Yacon syrup or stevia to taste (or choose from list of allowed sweeteners on page 228)

Add all ingredients to a blender. Blend until smooth.

Serves 2

Sesame Fish

½ cup tamari (gluten-free) sauce

2 teaspoons chopped garlic

2 tablespoons macadamia nut oil

1 teaspoon sesame oil

Pepper to taste

4 4-ounce sections of halibut

3 tablespoons sesame seeds

Heat oven to 400°F. In a small bowl, whisk together macadamia nut oil, sesame oil, tamari sauce, and pepper until well blended. Place the fish on a baking sheet. Pour tamari-sesame sauce over fish. Sprinkle sesame seeds evenly over fish. Bake for 15 minutes or until fish flakes easily with a fork.

Serves 4

Sausage, Spinach, and Cheese Egg Muffins

1 teaspoon extra-virgin olive oil to grease muffin tins

1 tablespoon extra-virgin olive oil for cooking

4 ounces ground turkey sausage

6 medium-size eggs, whisked completely

¼ cup medium chopped fresh spinach, packed tightly

¼ cup shredded cheddar cheese

⅛ teaspoon garlic powder
Salt and pepper

Heat oven to 325°F. In a muffin tin, use the oil to lightly grease each muffin cup. Heat a large skillet over medium heat. Add sausage and cook until sausage is browned. In a large bowl, combine eggs, sausage, spinach, cheese, garlic powder, and salt and pepper to taste. Pour egg mixture evenly into muffin cups. Cook for 20 minutes. Use a knife to loosen edges from pan to help with removal of the egg muffin.

Serves 6

Halibut Tacos

1 pound skinned and boned halibut, divided into four servings
1 tablespoon extra-virgin olive oil
1 avocado, pit removed and sliced
½ cup chopped cilantro
1 cup chopped tomatoes
½ cup chopped onion
Salsa to taste
Salt and pepper to taste
1 lemon, quartered
8 low-carb, high-fiber tortillas

Heat oil over medium-size skillet. Season fish pieces with salt and pepper. Cook fish for 10 minutes, turning fish over to brown both sides. Meanwhile heat tortillas in 300°F oven until warmed through. Lightly flake fish and add to tortilla. Top fish with 2 slices of avocado, cilantro, tomatoes, onion, and salsa. Serve with lemon wedge. Each serving is two tortillas.

Serves 4

Sautéed Spicy Green Beans

½ pound fresh green beans

2 tablespoons macadamia nut oil

3 garlic cloves, finely minced

1 teaspoon red pepper flakes (optional and to taste)

Salt and pepper to taste

Bring 2 cups of water to a boil. Add green beans. Reduce heat to medium and cook for 5 minutes. Drain beans and set aside. Heat a skillet over medium-high heat. Add garlic and red pepper flakes. Sauté for 1 minute or until fragrant. Add green beans, salt, and pepper. Mix very well.

Serves 2

FATflammation-Free Smoothie

1 cup green tea

1 cup spinach

½ cup blueberries

1 tablespoon chia seeds

½ teaspoon turmeric

½ teaspoon ginger

½ teaspoon cinnamon

Add all ingredients to a blender. Blend until smooth or desired consistency.

Serves 1

Chicken and Wild Rice Soup

1 tablespoon olive oil

1 red bell pepper chopped

2 celery stalks, chopped

2 garlic cloves, mashed

6 cups low-sodium chicken broth

1 pound diced chicken breast

¾ cup wild rice

Salt and pepper to taste

Heat oil in a large soup pot. Add garlic, bell pepper, and celery. Sauté until vegetables are softened. Add in chicken and sauté until lightly browned. Add the chicken broth, wild rice, and salt and pepper. Stir and bring to a boil. Reduce heat and simmer for 30 to 40 minutes or until the rice is done.

Serves 6

Roast Turkey Thighs with Herbs

2 pounds skinless, boneless turkey thighs

2 tablespoons macadamia nut oil

1 teaspoon garlic powder

1 teaspoon dried thyme

1 teaspoon dried sage

½ cup water or chicken broth

Salt and pepper to taste

Heat oven to 400°F. Rub oil over turkey thighs. Season thighs with garlic powder, thyme, sage, and salt and pepper. Add ½ cup of water or chicken broth to roasting pan. Place thighs in pan and roast for 35 to 40 minutes. Turn thighs and cook for another 30 minutes or until inserted meat thermometer reads 165°F.

Serves 3–4

Quick Breakfast Burrito

½ tablespoon grass-fed butter

1 strip turkey bacon

1 medium-size egg

¼ cup reduced-fat shredded cheese

1 low-carb whole-grain tortilla

¼ avocado, sliced

Salt and pepper

In a medium-size pan, melt butter. Add bacon and cook until desired doneness. Add eggs and scramble; salt and pepper to taste. Place the cooked eggs on the tortilla. Top eggs with avocado and bacon slices. Sprinkle cheese on top. Roll up each side of the tortilla and serve.

Serves 1

Quick Black Bean Burger

1 15-ounce can black beans, rinsed and drained

½ cup chopped onion

1 whole medium-size egg, whisked well

1 teaspoon finely minced garlic

1 teaspoon chili powder

⅛ teaspoon turmeric

Salt and pepper to taste

1 tablespoon extra-virgin olive oil

Sliced onion

Sliced tomato

Lettuce

3 tablespoons guacamole

3 sprouted "thin-style" burger buns (or substitute with
    lettuce wrap of choice)

In a large mixing bowl, add black beans. Mash beans well with a fork. Add in onion, egg, garlic, chili powder, turmeric, and salt and pepper. Mix well. Shape into patties. Heat the oil in large skillet over medium heat. Add patties and cook until browned on both sides. If desired, toast buns. Place patty on bun. Top patties with tomato, onion, lettuce, and guacamole. (You can freeze patties to be reheated at another time.)

Serves 3

Sautéed Garlic Sea Scallops

3 tablespoons macadamia nut oil
16 sea scallops
½ cup almond flour
3 garlic cloves, finely minced
½ cup parsley, chopped
2 tablespoons lemon juice
Salt and pepper to taste

Heat oil in a large skillet over medium-high heat. Meanwhile roll scallops in almond flour. Add garlic to the pan and cook until fragrant about 1 minute. Add scallops. Brown scallops and cook about 2 minutes on each side, depending on size. When scallops are opaque and tender, remove and keep warm. Add parsley and lemon juice to the pan. Bring to a quick simmer. Return the scallops to the skillet. Add salt and pepper and heat through. Serve immediately.

Serves 4

MORE RECIPES

Salads: What You Need To Know

Not only are salads delicious and easy to make, they are also anti-inflammatory.

Look at the recipes and lists below to get some ideas of how you can mix and match to create your own signature salad. Experiment with different tastes. If you have never put berries in your salad, for example, try it. You might love it! Each ingredient has different phytonutrients that confer anti-inflammatory and fat-melting benefits, so variety is important. To get as many nutrients as possible, try to "eat the rainbow" of vegetables and fruits. Just remember that greens and fresh vegetables tend to stay fresh for a very short time. Buy enough to last three or four days. Then you need to head back to the store. Also don't forget about the possibility of adding some protein to your salads in the form of beans or other legumes. A small green salad with beans makes a great FATflammation-free snack!

Don't be afraid to be creative and find some new combinations. To help with a busy schedule, you can also purchase veggies and salad greens cut up and ready to throw together. The darker the greens, the healthier, so steer away from the iceberg lettuce as it has virtually no FATflammation-free benefits.

If you would like to create a main meal out of a salad, add a lean protein, and increase the amount of veggies, and you will have super health in a bowl.

Here are some basic salad recipes for you to try. Each salad recipe below serves one. Use 1 to 2 teaspoons of vinaigrette for each portion of a side salad. If you are making a main dish salad, use 1 to 2 tablespoons of vinaigrette.

Small Baby Spinach Salad

1 big handful of baby spinach leaves
½ cup sliced cucumber
½ cup grape or cherry tomatoes, halved
1 tablespoon red onion
Salt and freshly ground black pepper to taste

Mix spinach, cucumber, tomatoes, red onion, and salt and pepper with your choice of Basic Vinaigrette (see recipe at end of salad recipes), vinaigrette of choice, or lemon juice with 1 to 2 teaspoons of extra-virgin olive oil.

Small Chopped Kale Salad

1 big handful of kale
1 tablespoon red onion
1 tablespoon chopped roasted red pepper
Salt and freshly ground pepper to taste

Mix kale, red onion, roasted red pepper, and salt and pepper with your choice of Basic Vinaigrette, vinaigrette of choice, or lemon juice with 1 to 2 teaspoons extra-virgin olive oil.

Small Chopped Romaine Salad

1 large handful of chopped or torn romaine lettuce
½ cup cherry tomatoes, halved
2 green onions or scallions, sliced
½ cup chopped red bell pepper
1 tablespoon fresh basil, chopped
Salt and freshly ground black pepper to taste

Mix romaine lettuce, tomatoes, green onions, red bell pepper, basil, and salt and pepper with your choice of Basic Vinaigrette, vinaigrette of choice, or lemon juice with 1 to 2 teaspoons olive oil.

Small Arugula and Butter Lettuce Salad

> 1 large handful of mixed arugula and butter leaf lettuce
> ½ cup artichoke hearts
> ¼ cup sliced mushrooms, raw
> 1 tablespoon roasted red pepper, chopped
> Salt and freshly ground black pepper to taste

Mix arugula, butter lettuce, artichoke hearts, roasted red pepper, mushrooms, and salt and pepper with your choice of Basic Vinaigrette, vinaigrette of choice or lemon juice with 1 to 2 teaspoons olive oil.

Small Spinach Salad with Red Bell Peppers and Red Onions

> 1 large handful of spinach leave
> ¼ cup diced red bell peppers
> ¼ cup sliced red onion
> Salt and freshly ground black pepper to taste

Mix spinach, red bell peppers, sliced red onion; season with salt and pepper and add your choice of Basic Vinaigrette, vinaigrette of choice, or lemon juice with 1 to 2 teaspoons olive oil.

Small "Any Green" Salad with Blueberries and Mint

> 1 large handful of leafy greens of choice
> ¼ cup blueberries

¼ cup diced red onion

1 tablespoon chopped mint

Salt and freshly ground black pepper to taste

Mix leafy greens, blueberries, diced red onion, mint; season with salt and pepper and add your choice of Basic Vinaigrette, vinaigrette of choice, or lemon juice with 1 to 2 teaspoons olive oil.

Small Spicy Watercress, Avocado, and Arugula Salad with Strawberries

1 large handful of watercress and arugula greens

1 tablespoon diced avocado

¼ cup sliced strawberries

¼ cup sliced red onion

Salt and freshly ground black pepper to taste

Mix watercress, arugula, avocado, strawberries, and red onion; season with salt and pepper and add your choice of Basic Vinaigrette, vinaigrette of choice, or lemon juice with 1 to 2 teaspoons olive oil.

Small Spinach Salad with Cannellini Beans

1 large handful of spinach leave

¼ cup of cannellini beans, rinsed and drained

¼ cup roasted red bell peppers

¼ cup sliced green onions

Salt and freshly ground black pepper to taste

Mix spinach, cannellini beans, roasted red bell peppers, and green onions; season with salt and pepper and add your choice of Basic Vinaigrette, vinaigrette of choice, or lemon juice with 1 to 2 teaspoons olive oil.

Small Arugula-Blueberry Salad with Garbanzo Beans

1 large handful of arugula
¼ cup of garbanzo beans
¼ cup fresh blueberries
1 tablespoon chopped chives
Salt and freshly ground black pepper to taste

Mix arugula, garbanzo beans, blueberries, and chives; season with salt and pepper and add your choice of Basic Vinaigrette, vinaigrette of choice, or lemon juice with 1 to 2 teaspoons olive oil.

Small Salad of Mixed Baby Greens and Bell Peppers

1 large handful of mixed baby greens
½ cup mix of chopped red, yellow, and green bell peppers
¼ cup sliced green onions
1 tablespoon blueberries
Salt and freshly ground pepper to taste

Mix baby greens, bell peppers, green onions, and blueberries; season with salt and pepper and add your choice of Basic Vinaigrette, vinaigrette of choice, or lemon juice with 1 to 2 teaspoons olive oil.

Chopped Green Salad with Broccoli Florets and Cherry Tomatoes

1 large handful combination of chopped romaine and collard greens
½ cup cherry or grape tomatoes, halved
¼ cup broccoli florets
¼ cup sliced green onions
1 teaspoon chia seeds
Salt and freshly ground black pepper to taste

Mix romaine/collard greens, tomatoes, broccoli florets, green onions, and chia seeds; season with salt and pepper and add your choice of Basic Vinaigrette, vinaigrette of choice, or lemon juice with 1 to 2 teaspoons olive oil.

Super easy-to-make vinaigrettes are also superhealthy! Make these delicious dressings ahead of time so you will have them on hand at a moment's notice.

Basic Vinaigrette

¾ cup extra-virgin olive oil
¼ cup red wine vinegar
Sea salt to taste
Freshly ground pepper to taste

In a bowl, whisk all ingredients together until emulsified. Refrigerate to store.

Balsamic Vinaigrette

¾ cup extra-virgin olive oil
¼ cup balsamic vinegar
1 teaspoon prepared Dijon mustard (not powdered)
Salt to taste
Freshly ground pepper to taste

In a bowl, whisk all ingredients together until emulsified. Refrigerate to store.

Classic Lemon Vinaigrette

3 tablespoons lemon juice
¾ cup extra-virgin olive oil
1 teaspoon prepared Dijon mustard (not powdered)
Sea salt to taste
Freshly ground pepper to taste

In a bowl, whisk all ingredients together until emulsified. Refrigerate to store.

Optional additions for salad dressings: Teaspoon of minced shallots, minced garlic, minced fresh herbs, teaspoon of any dried herbs.

Basic Salad Green Choices

Arugula

Asparagus tips

Beet greens

Bell peppers (red, green, yellow, purple, and roasted)

Bibb lettuce

Bok choy

Broccoli florets

Butter leaf lettuce

Cauliflower florets

Cheese (feta, chevre, shaved parmesan, shredded low-fat cheese)

Collard greens

Dandelion greens

Endive

Escarole

Herbs (mint, basil, oregano)

Kale and baby kale

Mixed herb salad greens

Mustard greens

Radicchio

Red leaf lettuce

Roasted red peppers

Romaine lettuce

Spinach

Turnip greens

Watercress

List of Salad Ingredients

Lean proteins such as eggs (1), nuts (1 T), seeds (1 T), tuna, salmon, shrimp, chicken, turkey or lean beef (4 ounces) (Note: Added protein, cheese, nuts are only for a whole meal salad.)

Artichoke hearts (packed in water—¼ cup)

Anchovies

Asparagus

Avocado (¼ of a small avocado)

Beans

Berries (blueberries, strawberries)

Bean sprouts

Bell peppers—red, orange, yellow, and green

Broccoli

Cauliflower

Celery

Cucumber

Garlic

Ginger

Jicama

Mushrooms (shitake, porcini, portobello, brown, button)

Nuts (pine nuts, walnuts, almonds, pistachios)

Olives

Onions—all varieties

Parsley

Pickled veggies (cultured)

Radishes

Roasted red peppers (packed in water)

Shallots

Summer squash

Tomatoes

Grape tomatoes

Zucchini

List of Salad Dressing Ingredients

Balsamic vinegar

Red wine vinegar

Lemon juice

Lime juice

Extra-virgin olive oil

Macadamia nut oil

Sesame oil

Dijon mustard

Pico de gallo

Salsa

EAT YOUR VEGGIES—STEAMED

Steaming is a superhealthy way to add more FATflammation-free veggies to your diet; it takes only minutes and is easy cleanup! Steaming is one of the best ways to cook vegetables because it retains nutrients that can easily be destroyed when you boil veggies.

There are two easy ways to steam vegetables.

Steaming Basket

In a large pot, add one or two inches of water or broth at the bottom of the pot. Add veggies such as cauliflower or broccoli to a steamer basket, place the lid on the pot (the lid should not cover the pot completely), and steam the veggies until crisp tender or to desired tenderness—3 to 5 minutes.

Pan Steaming

Make sure your pan is large enough to hold veggies such as broccoli or cauliflower in one layer. Add ½ to 1 inch of water or broth to pan. When the water or broth comes to a boil, add veggies, place lid on pot allowing for ventilation and steam until veggies are crisp tender or to desired doneness—3 to 5 minutes. Keep an eye on the water level as it can evaporate quickly and require additional water or broth.

Once your veggies are done, you can add a 1 teaspoon drizzle of anti-inflammatory extra-virgin olive oil, macadamia nut oil, or coconut oil. Adding a healthy fat will help your body absorb nutrients to reverse FATflammation. Also add lemon juice or garlic; toss veggies with 1 teaspoon of pesto or 1 teaspoon of your own homemade vinaigrette with herbs and spices of choice. For example, steamed asparagus is excellent with drizzled olive oil and a squeeze of lemon juice.

Best Veggies to Steam

Asparagus	Red pepper slices
Artichokes	Spinach
Broccoli	Steamed vegetable medley
Bok choy	Summer squash
Chinese broccoli	Winter squash such as
Cauliflower	butternut, acorn
Green beans	Zucchini

EAT YOUR VEGGIES—SAUTÉED

Here's another way to add more FATflammation-fighting nutrients, phyto-chemicals, and fiber to your diet. Whenever possible, try to find fresh seasonal local veggies that will give you more nutritional bang for your buck. Frozen is another excellent choice as all produce is frozen at the peak of freshness.

Dry Sautéed Leafy Greens

If you are going to sauté green leafy veggies such as spinach or kale, simply rinse them and place in pan. The moisture from the leafy greens will help them cook without added oil. Keep an eye on the pot to make sure that all the water doesn't evaporate. When the greens are sautéed to your liking, place them on a plate and drizzle or add 1 teaspoon of olive oil.

Sautéed Veggies

Before cooking, heat pan to medium-high heat. You can use water or low-sodium chicken broth. Make sure all veggies are uniformly diced or chopped to facilitate even cooking. Add veggies, garlic, onions, herbs, spices, salt, or pepper to the pan and stir frequently until cooked through. When finished, drizzle with 1 teaspoon extra-virgin olive, macadamia nut, sesame, or coconut oil. Think about adding in other ingredients such as ginger, turmeric, cumin, cayenne pepper, mushrooms, or minced fresh herbs such as oregano, thyme, or cilantro.

If you are sautéing more than one type of veggie, the harder and denser veggie will require more cooking time. Cook the harder veggie first until crisp tender, then add in the remaining veggie(s).

Best Veggies to Sauté

Asparagus	Kale
Bell peppers (red, yellow, orange, green)	Leafy greens (all varieties)
	Mushrooms (all varieties)
Broccoli	Onions
Broccoli rabe	Radishes
Brussels sprouts, chopped	Red chard
Cabbage, shredded	Snow peas
Cauliflower	Spinach
Cherry tomatoes	Summer quash
Celery	Water chestnuts
Green beans	Zucchini

Sautéed Spinach and Kale

Add 2 tablespoons of low-sodium chicken broth to medium-hot skillet large enough to hold veggies. Add 1 teaspoon finely minced garlic, a pinch of red pepper flakes, 1 teaspoon dried basil, and salt and pepper to taste. Simmer until garlic is aromatic. Add to the pan 1½ cups spinach, 1 cup kale, and sauté until greens are wilted and all ingredients are combined. When spinach and kale are wilted and cook to your desired taste, place on a plate and drizzle or add 1 teaspoon of olive, macadamia nut, sesame, or coconut oil.

Serves 1–2

Sautéed Zucchini

Add 2 tablespoons low-sodium chicken broth to a medium-hot skillet large enough to hold 2 sliced zucchinis. When chicken broth is hot, add 1 teaspoon of minced garlic and simmer until aromatic. Add zucchini, salt and pepper to taste, and sauté until done. When zucchini is ready, drizzle or add 1 teaspoon of olive, macadamia nut, or coconut oil.

Serves 1–2

Quick Vegetable Sauté

Add 2 tablespoon low-sodium chicken broth to a medium-hot pan large enough to hold veggies. Add 1 tablespoon of minced shallot or garlic and 4 cups frozen veggies. Stir until veggies are tender. Add in salt, pepper, and herbs of choice. Drizzle each serving with 1 teaspoon of olive, macadamia nut, sesame, or coconut oil.

Serves 4

More Ideas for Snacks

After you've completed three weeks of the FATflammation-Free Diet Program, you can become a little more adventurous with your snacks. By now you should have a pretty good grasp of what you should and shouldn't be eating. Every now and then, you can even indulge in a little dark chocolate. Try some of the following ideas:

Crispy cheese crackers: slice string cheese crossways into medallions, then melt in 325°F oven until golden and crispy.

Mary's Gone Crackers (gluten free) with black bean, hummus, or lentil dip. (See Dip Recipes.)

4 ounces of plain unsweetened coconut yogurt mixed with defrosted raspberries (and juice) along with choice of nuts.

Sliced meat wrapped around a cheese stick.

Celery sticks with lower-fat cream cheese.

Lemony avocado endive boats: mash ⅓ avocado, add lemon juice and pepper to taste—fill endive leaves.

Five halved cherry tomatoes with 2 tablespoons of fresh goat cheese or low-fat ricotta cheese. Sprinkle with herb of choice such as basil.

Cook 14 frozen sweet potato fries according to package instructions; mix 2 tablespoons of plain nonsweetened yogurt with 2 teaspoons chipotle sauce for dipping.

Cauliflower Popcorn (See Snack Recipes.)

Krispy Kale Chips (See Snack Recipes.)

¼ cup freeze-dried berries and 3 walnut halves.

½ baked apple with 1 teaspoon coconut butter, sprinkled with cinnamon.

Combine and mix ¼ cup unsalted roasted nuts of choice and 1 ounce melted dark chocolate (70% to 80% cacao). Drop onto wax paper; refrigerate until set.

Chocolate milk: mix together 2 tablespoons chocolate stevia-sweetened whey protein and 6 ounces almond milk.

SNACK RECIPES

Cauliflower Popcorn

1 head cauliflower, cut into small florets
4 tablespoons olive oil
Salt to taste

Heat oven to 425°F. In a large bowl combine cauliflower, olive oil, and salt. Mix well. Transfer cauliflower onto a baking sheet. Roast until browned and a bit crispy, turning halfway through cooking, about 30 minutes.

Krispy Kale Chips

1 bunch of kale, washed and dried thoroughly
Olive oil
Salt to taste

Heat oven to 350°F. With a knife, remove the thick rib from the kale leaves. Tear the kale into bite-sized pieces. Place kale on baking sheet. Drizzle with oil and coat leaves well. Add salt. Bake until crisp, about 15 minutes.

DIP RECIPES

Black Bean Dip

2 15-ounce cans of black beans, rinsed and drained
½ cup chopped onion
1 clove garlic, minced

1 small jalapeño, seeded and minced

¼ cup chopped cilantro

2 tablespoons lime juice

1 teaspoon ground cumin

1 teaspoon chili powder

Salt and freshly ground pepper to taste

Put all ingredients into a blender or food processor. Blend until creamy smooth. Place in a serving bowl. Cover and refrigerate until ready to use.

Hummus Dip

1 15-ounce can garbanzo beans (chickpeas), rinsed and drained

3 tablespoons lemon juice

3 tablespoons tahini

2 cloves garlic, crushed

½ teaspoon sea salt

2 tablespoons extra-virgin olive oil

Put all ingredients into a blender or food processor. Blend until creamy smooth. Place in serving bowl. Cover and refrigerate until ready to use.

Lentil Dip

1 15-ounce can lentils, rinsed and drained

2 cloves of garlic, peeled and crushed

1 tablespoon lime juice

2 tablespoons olive oil

Salt and freshly ground pepper to taste

Put all ingredients into a blender or food processor. Blend until creamy smooth. Place in a serving bowl. Cover and refrigerate until ready to use.

END NOTE TO READERS

In our quest to lose weight, we sometimes focus only on the pounds or inches lost. Yes, our primary goal has been to lose weight. But it's my fervent hope that in the process of reversing the inflammation in your fat cells, you are now beginning to understand what optimal health feels like.

I hope all the new information you've received will help you transition to a lifetime of healthy choices. The FATflammation-Free Diet Program has given you tools to help you continue your lifelong journey, but only you are responsible for your weight loss and only you are in control of the next chapter of your life.

You have learned what it takes to reduce inflamed fat cells. Please do continue to be proactive in all your health and weight-loss choices. To really come full circle, I'd like to suggest that you pass on what you have learned to others. My goal has always been to help others, and I would like you to share that goal. By educating others, you learn twice—by first going through it yourself and by then teaching others what you have learned. This is true empowerment.

ACKNOWLEDGMENTS

I am truly fortunate to have such an exceptional team surrounding me at HarperOne. Every step of the way, this project was filled with team excellence and kind support in making this book a reality. Thank you to the entire HarperCollins organization for your belief in the book.

I would like to express my deepest, sincerest, heartfelt gratitude to Julia Coopersmith, whose untiring enthusiasm, excellence, hard work, and endless hours of dedication and friendship helped me share my message.

My sincere gratitude to my agent and friend Eileen Cope, who saw my vision and without whom this book would not have been written.

My deepest thanks to my editor, Gideon Weil, for his enthusiasm, patience, creative abilities, and support.

Gratitude and appreciation to Miles Doyle, my developmental editor, for his creative ability, flexibility, and long hours.

Thank you to marketing director Amy VanLangen for her acumen, kindness, and energy.

My sincere gratitude to Melinda Mullin, publicity director, for her enthusiastic and unwavering support.

Thank you Natalie Blachere, production editor, and Laurie McGee, copy editor, for all your excellent skills and painstaking work.

Thank you to Hilary Lawson for her assistance whenever needed.

I would like to thank my original editor Nancy Hancock for her enthusiasm and belief in the creation of this book.

My indebtedness, gratitude, and appreciation to my manager, Robert L. Choat, Ph.D., who has been a source of continual steadfast support and patience.

Thanks also to my wonderful friends who have supported me during the creation of this book completely.

I would like to thank my beautiful and supportive family—my father Wayne Rickert, my brothers Mark, Lance, and Scott, and my sister Dawn.

And last, but absolutely not least, I would also like to acknowledge with love and gratitude, my husband Albert Shemek for his continuous support in so many ways during the creation of this book. It is true that actions speak louder than words.

And let's not forget Skye, whose fuzzy presence always brightens my life.

Chapter One: Why Cutting Calories Doesn't Cut It

Chilton, Floyd, et. al. "Mechanisms by Which Botanical Lipids Affect Inflammatory Disorders." *American Journal of Clinical Investigation* 87 (2008): 4985–5035. ajcn.nutrition.org/content/87/2/498S.full.

The Christian Broadcasting Network. "A Silent Killer in Our Midst." www.cbn.com/health/naturalhealth/drsears_silentkiller.aspx.

Cildir, Gökhan, Semih Can Akincilar, and Vinay Tergaonkar. "Chronic Adipose Tissue Inflammation: All Immune Cells on the Stage." *Trends in Molecular Medicine* 19 (2013): 487–500. doi:10.1016/j.molmed.2013.05.001.

Coppack, Simon W. "Pro-inflammatory Cytokines and Adipose Tissue." *Proceedings of the Nutrition Society* 60 (2001): 349–356. doi:10.1079/PNS2001110.

Egger, Garry. "Obesity, Chronic Disease, and Economic Growth: A Case for 'Big Picture' Prevention." *Advances in Preventative Medicine* 2011 (2011): 1–6. doi:10.4061/2011/149158.

Greenberg, Andrew S., and Martin S. Obin. "Obesity and the Role of Adipose Tissue in Inflammation and Metabolism." *American Journal of Clinical Nutrition* 83 (2006): 461S–465S. ajcn.nutrition.org/content/83/2/461S.full.

Gregor, Margaret F., and Gökhan S. Hotamisligil. "Inflammatory Mechanisms in Obesity." *Annual Review of Immunology* 29 (2011): 415–445. doi:10.1146/annurev-immunol-031210-101322.

Horng, Tiffany, and Gökhan S. Hotamisligil. "Linking the Inflammasome to Obesity-Related Disease." *Nature Medicine* 17 (2011): 164–165. 211.144.68.84:9998/91keshi/Public/File/39/17–2/pdf/nm0211–164.pdf.

Johnson, Amy R., J. Justin Milner, and Liza Makowski. "The Inflammation Highway: Metabolism Accelerates Inflammatory Traffic in Obesity." *Immunological Reviews* 249 (2012): 218–238. doi:10.1111/j.1600–065X.2012.01151.x.

Lumeng, Cary N., and Alan R. Saltiel. "Inflammatory Links Between Obesity and Metabolic Disease." *Journal of Clinical Investigation* 121 (2011): 2111–2117. doi:10.1172/JCI57132.

Mayo Clinic. "What Is New in Adipose Tissue?" www.mayoclinic.org/medical-professionals/clinical-updates/endocrinology/what-new-adipose-tissue.

McArdle, Maeve A., Orla M. Finucane, Ruth M. Connaughton, Aoibheann M. McMorrow, and Helen M. Roche. "Mechanisms of Obesity-Induced Inflammation and Insulin Resistance:

Insights into the Emerging Role of Nutritional Strategies." *Frontiers in Endocrinology* 4 (2013): 1–23 . doi:10.3389/fendo.2013.00052.

Methodist Hospital, Houston. "Obesity Makes Fat Cells Act Like They're Infected." *ScienceDaily.* www.sciencedaily.com/releases/2013/03/130305145145.htm.

Nishimura, Satoshi, Ichiro Manabe, and Ryozo Nagai. "Adipose Tissue Inflammation in Obesity and Metabolic Syndrome." *Discovery Medicine* 17 (2014). www.discoverymedicine.com/Satoshi-Nishimura/2009/09/22/adipose-tissue-inflammation-in-obesity-and-metabolic-syndrome/.

Pandey, A. K., G. Pandey, S. S. Pandey, and B. L. Pandey. "Human Biology of Diet and Lifestyle Linked Chronic Inflammatory Non-Communicable Disease Epidemic—A Review." *Human Biology Review* 3 (2014): 25–42.

Paresh Dandona, Ahmad Aljada, and Arindam Bandyopadhyay. "Inflammation: The Link Between Insulin Resistance, Obesity and Diabetes." *Trends in Immunology* 25 (2004): 4–7. doi:10.1016/j.it.2003.10.013.

Science Codex. "Body Fat Stored in the Liver, Not the Belly, Is the Best Indicator of Disease." www.sciencecodex.com/fat_in_the_liver_not_the_belly_is_a_better_marker_for_disease_risk.

Sears, Barry. *Toxic Fat.* Nashville: Thomas Nelson, 2008.

Sun, Shengyi, Yewei Ji, Sander Kersten, and Lind Qi. "Mechanisms of Inflammatory Responses in Obese Adipose Tissue." *Annual Review of Nutrition* 32 (2012): 261–286. doi:10.1146/annurev-nutr-071811-150623.

University of Texas Health Science Center at Houston. "First Link Found Between Obesity, Inflammation and Vascular Disease." *ScienceDaily.* www.sciencedaily.com/releases/2005/09/050917085024.htm.

Wellen, Kathryn E., and Gökhan S. Hotamisligil. "Obesity-Induced Inflammatory Changes in Adipose Tissue." *Journal of Clinical Investigation* 112 (2003): 1785–1788. doi:10.1172/JCI20514.

Wisse, Brent E. "The Inflammatory Syndrome: The Role of Adipose Tissue Cytokines in Metabolic Disorders Linked to Obesity." *Frontiers in Nephrology* 15 (2004): 2792–2800. doi:10.1097/01.ASN.0000141966.69934.21.

Xu, H., et. al. "Chronic Inflammation in Fat Plays a Crucial Role in the Development of Obesity-Related Insulin Resistance." *Journal of Clinical Investigation* 112 (2003): 1821–1830. doi:10.1172/JCI19451.

Zhang, W.-J., L.-L. Chen, J. Zheng, L. Lin, J.-Y. Zhang, and X. Hu. "Association of Adult Weight Gain and Nonalcoholic Fatty Liver in a Cross-Sectional Study in Wan Song Community, China." *Brazilian Journal of Medical and Biological Research* 47 (2014). doi:10.1590/1414-431X20133058.

Ziccardi, Patrizia, Francesco Nappo, Giovanni Giugliano, et al. "Reduction of Inflammatory Cytokine Concentrations and Improvement of Endothelial Functions in Obese Women After Weight Loss Over One Year." *Circulation* 105 (2002): 804–809. doi:10.1161/hc0702.104279.

Chapter Two: Are You Overfed and Undernourished?

Damms-Machado, Antje, Gesine Weser, and Stephan C. Bischoff. "Micronutrient Deficiency in Obese Subjects Undergoing Low Calorie Diet." *Nutrition Journal* 11, no. 34 (2012): 1–10. doi:10.1186/1475-2891-11-34.

Garcia, Olga P., Kurt Z. Long, and Jorge L. Rosado. "Impact of Micronutrient Deficiencies on Obesity." *Nutrition Reviews* 67 (2009): 559–572. doi:10.1111/j.1753-4887.2009.00228.x.

University of Florida. "Phytochemicals in Plant-based Foods Could Help Battle Obesity, Disease." *ScienceDaily*. www.sciencedaily.com/releases/2009/10/091021144251.htm.

Zhu, Haidong, Matthew Belcher, and Pim van der Harst. "Healthy Aging and Disease: Role for Telomere Biology?" *Clinical Science* 120 (2011): 427–440. doi:10.1042/CS20100385.

Chapter Three: Fat: Three Little Letters That Carry a Lot of Weight

Chandran, Manju, Theodore Ciaraldi, Susan A. Phillips, and Robert R. Henry. "Adiponectin: More Than Just Another Fat Cell Hormone?" *Diabetes Care* 26 (2003): 2442–2450. doi:10.2337/diacare.26.8.2442.

Choi, Sang-Woon, and Simonetta Friso. "Epigenetics: A New Bridge Between Nutrition and Health." *Advances in Nutrition* 1 (2010): 8–16. doi:10.3945/an.110.1004.

Dolinoy, Dana C. "The Agouti Mouse Model: An Epigenetic Biosensor for Nutritional and Environmental Alterations on the Fetal Epigenome." *Nutrition Review* 66 (2008): S7–S11. doi:10.1111/j.1753-4887.2008.00056.x.

Endocrine Society. "Appetite Hormone Misfires in Obese People." *ScienceDaily*. www.sciencedaily.com/releases/2013/08/130820134753.html.

Experience Life. "Functional Wellness, Part 2: Hormones and Inflammation." experiencelife.com/article/functional-wellness-part-2-hormones-and-inflammation/.

Herrera, Blanca M., Sarah Keildson, and Cecilia Lindgren. "Genetics and Epigenetics of Obesity." *Maturitas* 69 (2011): 41–49. doi:10.1016/j.maturitas.2011.02.018.

Life Extension Magazine. "Balancing Appetite Hormones to Reduce Hunger and Lose Weight." www.lef.org/magazine/mag2013/ss2013_Balancing-Appetite-Hormones-to-Reduce-Hunger-and-Lose-Weight_01.htm.

Martinez, J. Alfredo, Paúl Cordero, Javier Campión, and Fermin I. Milagro. "Interplay of Early-Life Nutritional Programming on Obesity, Inflammation and Epigenetic Outcomes." *Proceedings of the Nutrition Society* 71 (2012): 276–283. doi:10.1017/S0029665112000055.

Milagro, Fermin I., Javier Campión, Paúl Cordero, et al. "A Dual Epigenomic Approach for the Search of Obesity Biomarkers: DNA Methylation in Relation to Diet-Induced Weight Loss." *Journal of the Federation of American Societies for Experimental Biology* 25 (2011): 1378–1389. doi:10.1096/fj.10-170365.

Silva, Flavìa M., Jussara C. de Almeida, and Ana M. Feoli. "Effect of Diet on Adiponectin Levels in Blood." *Nutrition Reviews* 69 (2011): 599–612. doi:10.1111/j.1753-4887.2011.00414.x.

UT Southwestern Medical Center. "Study Unlocks Origin of Brown Fat Cells, Important in Weight Maintenance." *ScienceDaily*. www.sciencedaily.com/releases/2013/09/130926102259.htm.

Wang, Qiong A., Caroline Tao, Rana K. Gupta, and Philipp E. Scherer. "Tracking Adipogenesis During White Adipose Tissue Development, Expansion and Regeneration." *Nature Medicine* 19 (2013): 1338–1344. doi:10.1038/nm.3324.

Waterland, R. A. "Assessing the Effects of High Methionine Intake on DNA Methylation." *Journal of Nutrition* 136 (2006): 1706S–1710S.

Waterland, R. A., and R. L. Jirtle. "Transposable Elements: Targets for Early Nutritional Effects on Epigenetic Gene Regulation." *Molecular and Cellular Biology* 23 (2003): 5293–5300. doi:10.1128/MCB.23.15.5293–5300.2003.

Waterland, R. A., M. Travisano, K. G. Tahilani, M. T. Rached, and S. Mirza. "Methyl Donor Supplementation Prevents Transgenerational Amplification of Obesity." *International Journal of Obesity* 32 (2008): 1373–1379. doi:10.1038/ijo.2008.100.

Wolff, George L., Ralph L. Kodell, Stephen R. Moore, and Craig A. Cooney. "Maternal Epigenetics and Methyl Supplements Affect Agouti Gene Expression in Avy/a Mice ." *Journal of the Federation of American Societies for Experimental Biology* 12 (1998): 949–957.

Zhao, X., et al. "PPAR-a Activator Fenofibrate Increases Renal CYP-Derived Eicosanoid Synthesis and Improves Endothelial Dilator Function in Obese Zucker Rats." *American Journal of Physiology* 290 (2006): H2187–H2195. doi:10.1152/ajpheart.00937.2005

Chapter Four: Break Up with the FATflammation Four

Avena, Nicole M., Pedro Rada, and Bartley G. Hoebel. "Evidence for Sugar Addiction: Behavioral and Neurochemical Effects of Intermittent, Excessive Sugar Intake." *Neuroscience and Behavioral Reviews* 32 (2008): 20–39. doi:10.1016/j.neubiorev.2007.04.019.

Avena, Nicole M., Pedro Rada, and Bartley G. Hoebel. "Sugar and Fat Bingeing Have Notable Differences in Addictive-like Behavior." *Journal of Nutrition* 139 (2009): 623–628. doi:10.3945/1jn.108.097584.

Basciano, Heather, Lisa Federico, and Khosrow Adeli. "Fructose, Insulin Resistance, and Metabolic Dyslipidemia." *Nutrition & Metabolism* 2 (2005). doi:10.1186/1743-7075-2-5.

Bocarsly, Miriam E., Elyse S. Powell, Nicole M. Avena, and Bartley G. Hoebel. "High-Fructose Corn Syrup Causes Characteristics of Obesity in Rats: Increased Body Weight, Body Fat and Triglyceride Levels." *Pharmacology, Biochemistry, and Behavior* 97 (2010): 101–106. doi:10.1016/j.pbb.2010.02.012.

Fortuna, J. L. "Sweet Preference, Sugar Addiction and the Familial History of Alcohol Dependence: Shared Neural Pathways and Genes." *Journal of Psychoactive Drugs* 42 (2010): 147–151. www.ncbi.nlm.nih.gov/pubmed/20648910.

Fowler, Sharon P., et al. "Fueling the Obesity Epidemic? Artificially Sweetened Beverage Use and Long-Term Weight Gain." *Obesity* 16 (2008): 1894–1900. doi:10.1038/oby.2008.284.

Hu, Frank B. "Are Refined Carbohydrates Worse Than Saturated Fat?" *American Journal of Clinical Nutrition* 91 (2010): 1541–1542. doi:10.3945/ajcn.2010.29622.

Hu, Frank B. "Globalization of Diabetes." *Diabetes Care* 34 (2011): 1249–1257. doi:10.2337/dc11-0442.

Jakobsen, Marianne U., et al. "Intake of Carbohydrates Compared with Intake of Saturated Fatty Acids and Risk of Myocardial Infarction: Importance of the Glycemic Index." *American Journal of Clinical Nutrition* 91 (2010): 1764–1768. doi:10.3945/1ajcn.2009.29099.

Lowndes, Joshua, et al. "The Effects of Four Hypocaloric Diets Containing Different Levels of Sucrose or High Fructose Corn Syrup on Weight Loss and Related Parameters." *Nutrition Journal* 11 (2012). doi:10.1186/1475-2891-11-55.

Page, Kathleen A., et al. "Effects of Fructose vs Glucose on Regional Cerebral Blood Flow in Brain Regions Involved with Appetite and Reward Pathways." *JAMA: The Journal of the American Medical Association* 309 (2013): 63–70. doi:10.1001/jama.2012.116975.

The People's Chemist. "Splenda: The Artificial Sweetener That Explodes Internally." thepeopleschemist.com/splenda-the-artificial-sweetener-that-explodes-internally/.

Scientific American. "Carbs against Cardio: More Evidence That Refined Carbohydrates, Not Fats, Threaten the Heart." www.scientificamerican.com/article/carbs-against-cardio/.

Stice, Eric, Kyle S. Burger, and Sonja Yokum. "Relative Ability of Fat and Sugar Tastes to Activate Reward, Gustatory, and Somatosensory Regions." *American Journal of Clinical Nutrition* 98 (2013): 1377–1384. doi:10.3945/ajcn.113.069443.

Swithers, Susan E. "Artificial Sweeteners Produce the Counterintuitive Effect of Inducing Metabolic Derangements." *Trends in Endocrinology & Metabolism* 24 (2013): p431–441. doi:10.1016/j.tem.2013.05.005.

Vos, Miriam B., and Joel L. Lavine. "Dietary Fructose in Nonalcoholic Fatty Liver Disease." *Hepatology* 57 (2013) 2525–2531. doi:10.1002/hep.26299.

Yang, Quig. "Gain Weight by "Going Diet " Artificial Sweeteners and the Neurobiology of Sugar Cravings." *Yale Journal of Biology and Medicine* 83 (2010): 101–108. www.ncbi.nlm.nih.gov/pmc/articles/PMC2892765/.

Chapter Five: Burn Fat by Eating (the Right) Fat

Adam, O., et al. "Anti-inflammatory Effects of a Low Arachidonic Acid Diet and Fish Oil in Patients with Rheumatoid Arthritis." *Rheumatology International* 23 (2003): 27–36. www.ncbi.nlm.nih.gov/pubmed/12548439.

Authority Nutrition. "Are Vegetable and Seed Oils Bad for Your Health? A Critical Look." authority-nutrition.com/are-vegetable-and-seed-oils-bad/.

Calder, Philip C. "N{dec45}3 Polyunsaturated Fatty Acids, Inflammation, and Inflammatory Diseases." *American Journal of Clinical Nutrition* 83 (2006): 1505S–1519S. ajcn.nutrition.org/content/83/6/S1505.full.

Dwyer, James H., Hooman Allayee, Kathleen M. Dwyer, et al. "Arachidonate 5-Lipoxygenase Promoter Genotype, Dietary Arachidonic Acid, and Atherosclerosis." *New England Journal of Medicine* 350 (2004): 29–37. keck.usc.edu/en/Research/Umbrella_Programs/Institute_for_Genetic_Medicine/IGM_Research_Units/IGM_Genetic_Faculty/~/media/Docs/Research/Dwyer%20 5-LO%20NEJM%202004.pdf.

Flores-Mateo, Gemma, et al. "Nut Intake and Adiposity: Meta-Analysis of Clinical Trials." *American Journal of Clinical Nutrition* (2013): 1–10. doi:10.3945/ajcn.111.031484.

Harvard School of Public Health. "Omega-3 Fatty Acids: An Essential Contribution." www.hsph.harvard.edu/nutritionsource/omega-3-fats/.

Life Extension. "Omega-7 Fatty Acids Decrease Hunger." blog.lef.org/2013/04/omega-7-fatty-acids-decrease-hunger.html.

Life Extension Blog. "Do Vegetable Oils Cause Heart Disease?" blog.lef.org/2013/03/vegetable-oils-cause-heart-disease.html

Massiera, Florence, Perla Saint-Marc, Josaine Seydoux, et al. "Arachidonic Acid and Prostacy-clin Signaling Promote Adipose Tissue Development: A Human Health Concern?" *Journal of Lipid Research* 44 (2003): 271–279. doi:10.1194/jlr.M200346-JLR200.

Messina, Mark, and Geoffrey Redmond. "Effects of Soy Protein and Soybean Isoflavones on Thyroid Function in Healthy Adults and Hypothyroid Patients: A Review of the Relevant Literature." *Thyroid* 16 (2006): 249–258. doi:10.1089/thy.2006.16.249.

Patterson, E., R. Wall, G. F. Fitzgerald, R. P. Ross, and C. Stanton, "Health Implications of High Dietary Omega-6 Polyunsaturated Fatty Acids." *Journal of Nutrition and Metabolism* 2012 (2012): 16 pages. http://www.hindawi.com/journals/jnme/2012/539426/. Doi:10.1155/2012/539426.

Sears, Barry. *Anti-Inflammatory Medicine: Dietary Modulation of Eicosanoids.* www.drsears.com/portals/6/documents/inflammation%20medical%20brochure.pdf.

Sears, Barry, and Camillo Ricordi. "Anti-Inflammatory Nutrition as a Pharmacological Approach to Treat Obesity." *Journal of Obesity* 2011 (2011): 1–14. doi:10.1155/2011/431985.

Siberian Tiger Naturals. "Omega–3 Fatty Acids and Health: An Overview." www.siberiantiger naturals.com/omega3.htm.

Wansink, Brian, and Pierre Chandon. "Can 'Low-Fat' Nutrition Labels Lead to Obesity?" *Journal of Marketing Research* 43 (2006): 605–617. doi: 10.1509/jmkr.43.4.605.

Weiler, H. A. "Dietary Supplementation of Arachidonic Acid Is Associated with Higher Whole Body Weight and Bone Mineral Density in Growing Pigs." *Pediatric Research* 47 (2000): 692–697. www.ncbi.nlm.nih.gov/pubmed/10813598.

Chapter Six: Beat Sluggish Metabolism, FATflammation's BFF

Astrup, Arne. "The Satiating Power of Protein—A Key to Obesity Prevention?" *American Journal of Clinical Nutrition* 82 (2005): 1–2. ajcn.nutrition.org/content/82/1/1.full.

Batterham, Marijka, et al. "High-Protein Meals May Benefit Fat Oxidation and Energy Expenditure in Individuals with Higher Body Fat." *Nutrition & Dietetics* 65 (2008): 246–252. doi:10.1111/j.1747-0080.2008.00311.x.

Henry, C. J., and B. Emery. "Effect of Spiced Food on Metabolic Rate." *Human Nutrition. Clinical Nutrition* 40 (1986): 165–168. www.ncbi.nlm.nih.gov/pubmed/3957721.

JAMA and Archives Journals. "When Overeating, Calories—Not Protein—Contribute to Increase in Body Fat, Study Finds." *ScienceDaily.* www.sciencedaily.com/releases/2012/01/120103165002.htm.

Leidy, Heather J., Laura C. Ortinau, Steve M. Douglas, and Heather A. Hoertel. "Beneficial Effects of a Higher-Protein Breakfast on the Appetitive, Hormonal, and Neural Signals Controlling Energy Intake Regulation in Overweight/Obese, 'Breakfast-Skipping,' Late-Adolescent Girls." *American Journal of Clinical Nutrition* 97 (2013): 677–688. doi: 10.3945/ajcn.112.053116.

Miller, Paige E., Dominik D. Alexander, and Vanessa Perez. "Effects of Whey Protein and Resistance Exercise on Body Composition: A Meta-Analysis of Randomized Controlled Trials." *Journal of the American College of Nutrition* 33 (2014): 163–175. doi:10.1080/07315724.2013.875365.

Vander Wal, J. S., A. Gupta, A. Khosla, and N. V. Dhurandhar. "Egg Breakfast Enhances Weight Loss." *International Journal of Obesity* 32 (2008): 1545–1551. doi:10.1038/ijo.2008.130.

Chapter Seven: Be Kind to Bugs

Ackerman, Jennifer. "How Bacteria in Our Bodies Protect Our Health." *Scientific American* 306 (2012): 37–43. www.scientificamerican.com/article/ultimate-social-network-bacteria-protects-health/.

AlterNet. "Mind-Gut Connection: Why Intestinal Bacteria May Have Important Effects on Your Brain." www.alternet.org/story/150783/mind-gut_connection%3A_why_intestinal_bacteria_may_have_important_effects_on_your_brain.

Asociación RUVID. "Alternative to Yogurt." *ScienceDaily.* www.sciencedaily.com/releases/2014/01/140103085356.htm.

Cantarel, Brandi L., Vincent Lombard, and Bernard Henrissat. "Complex Carbohydrate Utilization by the Healthy Human Microbiome." *PloS ONE* 7 (2012). doi:10.1371/journal.pone.0028742.

Chicago Tribune Lifestyles. "Feed Your 'Good' Bacteria." articles.chicagotribune.com/2012–07–11/features/sns-201207110900—tms—foodstylts—v-f20120711-20120711_1_friendly-bacteria-lactic-acid-bacteria-beneficial-bugs.

David, Lawrence A., et al. "Diet Rapidly and Reproducibly Alters the Human Gut Microbiome." *Nature* (2013). doi:10.1038/nature12820.

Delzenne, Nathalie M., Audrey M. Neyrinck, Fredrik Bäckhed, and Patrice D. Cani. "Targeting Gut Microbiota in Obesity: Effects of Prebiotics and Probiotics." *Nature Reviews Endocrinology* 7 (2011): 639–646. www.ucllouvain.be/cps/ucl/doc/ir-ldri/images/DelzenneNatRevEndocrinol2011.pdf.

Dr. Mercola.com. *Peak Fitness.* "How Probiotics May Aid Your Weight Management." fitness.mercola.com/sites/fitness/archive/2014/01/17/probiotics-weight-management.aspx.

Genta, Susana, Wilfredo Cabrera, Natalia Habib, et al. "Yacon Syrup: Beneficial Effects on Obesity and Insulin Resistance in Humans." *Clinical Nutrition* 28 (2009): 182–187. doi:10.1016/j.clnu.2009.01.013.

The Human Microbiome Project Consortium. "Structure, Function and Diversity of the Healthy Human Microbiome." *Nature* 486 (2012): 207–214. doi:10.1038/nature11234.

Kadooka, Yukio, et al. "Effect of *Lactobacillus gasseri* SBT2055 in Fermented Milk on Abdominal Adiposity in Adults in a Randomised Controlled Trial." *Human and Clinical Nutrition* 110 (2013): 1696–1703. doi:10.1017/S0007114513001037.

Kadooka, Yukio, et al. "Regulation of Abdominal Adiposity by Probiotics (*Lactobacillus gasseri* SBT2055) in Adults with Obese Tendencies in a Randomized Controlled Trial." *European Journal of Clinical Nutrition* 64 (2010): 636–643. doi:10.1038/ejcn.2010.19.

Krajmalnik-Brown, Rosa, Zehra-Esra Ilhan, Dae-Wook Kang, and John K. DiBaise. "Effects of Gut Microbes on Nutrient Absorption and Energy Regulation." *Nutrition in Clinical Practice: Official Publication of the American Society for Parenteral and Enteral Nutrition* 27 (2012): 201–214. doi:10.1177/0884533611436116.

Kresser, Chris. "A Healthy Gut Is the Hidden Key to Weight Loss." chriskresser.com/a-healthy-gut-is-the-hidden-key-to-weight-loss.

Lipman, Dr. Frank. "Probiotic Power: The Path to a Happy Belly Is Paved with Good Bacteria." www.drfranklipman.com/probiotic-power/.

NIH News. "NIH Human Microbiome Project Defines Normal Bacterial Makeup of the Body." *National Institutes of Health* (2012). www.genome.gov/27549144.

NIH Research Matters. "Gut Microbes and Diet Interact to Affect Obesity." *National Institutes of Health* (2013). www.nih.gov/researchmatters/september2013/09162013obesity.htm.

Pearson, Helen. "Fat People Harbour 'Fat' Microbes." *Nature News* (2006). doi:10.1038/news061218-6.

Robinson, Courtney J., Brendan J. M. Bohannan, and Vincent B. Young. "From Structure to Function: The Ecology of Host-Associated Microbial Communities." *Microbiology and Molecular Biology Reviews* 74 (2010): 453–476. doi:10.1128/MMBR.00014-10.

Université Laval. "Certain Probiotics Could Help Women Lose Weight, Study Finds." *ScienceDaily*. www.sciencedaily.com/releases/2014/01/140128103537.htm.

University of Iowa. "Bacteria and Fat: A 'Perfect Storm' for Inflammation." *ScienceDaily*. www.sciencedaily.com/releases/2013/10/131030185153.htm.

VIB. "Intestinal Flora Determines Health of Obese People." *ScienceDaily*. www.sciencedaily.com/releases/2013/08/130828131932.htm.

Chapter Eight: Beware the Bane of Grain

Aggarwal, Saurabh, Benjamin Lebwohl, and Peter H. R. Green. "Screening for Celiac Disease in Average-Risk and High-Risk Populations." *Therapeutic Advances in Gastroenterology* 5 (2012): 37–47. doi:10.1177/1756283X11417038.

Lipman, Dr. Frank. "Are Food Sensitivities Making You Fat and Sick? 7 Ways to Fight Back and Drop Weight Fast." www.drfranklipman.com/food-sensitivities-are-making-you-fat-and-sick/.

Westman, Eric C., et al. "Low-Carbohydrate Nutrition and Metabolism." *American Journal of Clinical Nutrition* 86 (2007): 276–284. ajcn.nutrition.org/content/86/2/276.full.

Chapter Nine: Starting a FATflammation-Free Life

Kaiser Permanente. "Keeping a Food Diary Doubles Diet Weight Loss, Study Suggests." *ScienceDaily*. www.sciencedaily.com/releases/2008/07/080708080738.htm.

Chapter Ten: Stock Your Kitchen with FATflammation-Free Food

Eder, K. "The Effects of a Dietary Oxidized Oil on Lipid Metabolism in Rats." *Lipids* 34 (1999): 717–725.

Geliebter, Allan, et al. "Overfeeding with Medium-Chain Triglyceride Diet Results in Diminished Deposition of Fat1–4." *American Journal of Clinical Nutrition* 37 (1983): 1–4. ajcn.nutrition.org/content/37/1/1.long.

Jacob, Alagée. "Coconut Oil—Learn More About This Superfood That Contains Healthful Saturated Fats." *Today's Dietician* 15 (2013): 56.

Liu, Yeou-Mei Christiana. "Medium-Chain Triglyceride (MCT) Ketogenic Therapy." *Epilepsia* 49 (2008): 33–36. doi:10.1111/j.1528-1167.2008.01830.

Lucas, Lisa, Aaron Russell, and Russell Keast. "Molecular Mechanisms of Inflammation. Anti-Inflammatory Benefits of Virgin Olive Oil and the Phenolic Compound Oleocanthal." *Current Pharmaceutical Design* 17 (2011): 754–768. doi:10.2174/138161211795428911.

St-Onge, M.-P., and P. J. H. Jones. "Greater Rise in Fat Oxidation with Medium-Chain Triglyceride Consumption Relative to Long-Chain Triglyceride Is Associated with Lower Initial Body Weight and Greater Loss of Subcutaneous Adipose Tissue." *International Journal of Obesity* 27 (2003): 1565–1571. doi:10.1038/sj.ijo.0802467.

Tsuzuki, Wakako, Akiko Matsuoka, and Kaori Ushida. "Formation of *Trans* Fatty Acids in Edible Oils During the Frying and Heating Process." *Food Chemistry* 123 (2010): 976–982. doi:10.1016/j.foodchem.2010.05.048.

Chapter Eleven: The FATflammation-Free Diet 3-Week Program

Anton, Stephen D., et al. "Effects of Chromium Picolinate on Food Intake and Satiety." *Diabetes Technology and Therapeutics* 10 (2008): 405–412. doi:10.1089/dia.2007.0292.

Doi, K. "Effect of Konjac Fibre (Glucomannan) on Glucose and Lipids." *European Journal of Clinical Nutrition* 49 (1995): S190–S197. www.ncbi.nlm.nih.gov/pubmed/8549522.

Fukushi, Yoshika, et al. "Lemon Polyphenols Suppress Diet-induced Obesity by Up-Regulation of mRNA Levels of the Enzymes Involved in â-Oxidation in Mouse White Adipose Tissue." *Journal of Clinical and Biochemical Nutrition* 43 (2008): 201–209. doi:10.3164/jcbn.2008066.

Keithley, Joyce, and Barbara Swanson. "Glucomannan and Obesity: A Critical Review." *Alternative Therapies* 11 (2005): 30–34. clinicalstudiespublishing.com/pdf/supplemental/Glucomannan_and_obesity_review.pdf.

Musso, Giovanni, Roberto Gambino, and Maurizio Cassader. "Obesity, Diabetes, and Gut Microbiota." *Diabetes Care* 33 (2010): 2277–2284. doi:10.2337/dc10-0556.

Östman, E. "Vinegar Supplementation Lowers Glucose and Insulin Responses and Increases Satiety After a Bread Meal in Healthy Subjects." *European Journal of Clinical Nutrition* 59 (2005): 983–988. doi:10.1038/sj.ejcn.1602197.

Sood, Nitesh, William L. Baker, and Craig I. Coleman. "Effect of Glucomannan on Plasma Lipid and Glucose Concentrations, Body Weight, and Blood Pressure: Systematic Review and Meta-Analysis." *American Journal of Clinical Nutrition* 88 (2008): 1167–1175. ajcn.nutrition.org/content/88/4/1167.full.

Vido, L., P. Facchin, I. Antonello, D. Gobber, and F. Rigon. "Childhood Obesity Treatment: Double Blinded Trial on Dietary Fibres (Glucomannan) Versus Placebo." *Pädiatrie and Pädologie* 28 (1993): 133–136. www.ncbi.nlm.nih.gov/pubmed/8247594.

Vuksan, V., D. J. Jenkins, P. Spadafora, et al. "Konjac-Mannan (Glucomannan) Improves Glycemia and Other Associated Risk Factors for Coronary Heart Disease in Type 2 Diabetes. A Randomized Controlled Metabolic Trial." *Diabetes Care* 22 (1999): 913–919. care.diabetesjournals.org/content/22/6/913.full.pdf.

Chapter Sixteen: It Takes More Than a Diet

Chaput, Jean Philippe, and Angelo Tremblay. "Adequate Sleep to Improve the Treatment of Obesity." *Canadian Medical Association Journal* 184 (2012): 1975–1976. doi:10.1503/cmaj.120876.

"Circuit Training," accessed April 25, 2014, http://www.brianmac.co.uk/circuit.html.

Daubenmeier, Jennifer, Jean Kristeller, Frederick M. Hecht, et al. "Mindfulness Intervention for Stress Eating to Reduce Cortisol and Abdominal Fat Among Overweight and Obese Women: An Exploratory Randomized Controlled Study." *Journal of Obesity* 2011 (2011): 13 pages. doi:10.1155/2011/651936.

Heart and Stroke Foundation of Canada. "High-Intensity Interval Training Combined with Mediterranean Diet Counselling 'Supersizes' Heart Health." *Canadian Cardiovascular Congress.* 2013. http://www.heartandstroke.com/site/apps/nlnet/content2.aspx?c=ikIQLcMWJtE&b=8846639&ct=13370183

Kaiser Permanente. "Keeping a Food Diary Doubles Diet Weight Loss, Study Suggests." *ScienceDaily.* www.sciencedaily.com/releases/2008/07/080708080738.htm.

Keller, Abiola. "Does the Perception That Stress Affects Health Matter? The Association with Health and Mortality." *Health Psychology* 31 (2012): 677–684. doi:10.1037/a0026743.

Klika, Brett, and Chris Jordan. "High-Intensity Circuit Training Using Body Weight: Maximum Results with Minimal Investment." *ACSM's Health & Fitness Journal* 17–3 (2009): 8–13, accessed April 25, 2014. doi: 10.1249/FIT.0b013e31828cb1e8.

Kong, Angela, Shirley A. A. Beresford, Catherine M. Alfano, et al. "Self-Monitoring and Eating-Related Behaviors Are Associated with 12-Month Weight Loss in Postmenopausal Overweight-to-Obese Women." *Journal of the Academy of Nutrition and Dietetics* 112 (2012): 1428–1435. doi:10.1016/j.jand.2012.05.014.

Kravitz, Len. "New Insights into Circuit Training," University of New Mexico website, accessed April 22, 2014, www.unm.edu/~lkravitz/Article%20folder/circuits05.html.

Kravitz, Len. "The Fitness Professional's Complete Guide to Circuits and Intervals," University of New Mexico website, accessed April 22, 2014, www.unm.edu/~lkravitz/Article%20folder/circuits.html.

Mercola.com. "8 Stress-Busting Tips from Experts." articles.mercola.com/sites/articles/archive/2013/11/07/8-stress-management-tips.aspx.

Montreal Heart Institute. "Interval Training and Healthy Eating Is Solution to Obesity, Study Shows." *ScienceDaily.* www.sciencedaily.com/releases/2011/04/110428101759.htm.

Peak Fitness. "The Importance of Intermittent Movement for Longevity." fitness.mercola.com/sites/fitness/archive/2013/12/13/sitting-standing-up.aspx.

Stokes, K. A., M. E. Nevill, G. M. Hall, and H. K. A. Lakomy. "The Time Course of the Human Growth Hormone Response to a 6 S and a 30 S Cycle Ergometer Sprint." *Journal of Sports Sciences* 20 (2002): 487–494. doi:10.1080/02640410252925152.

Stokes, K.A., Nevill, M.E., Hall, G.M. and Lakomy, H.K. "The time course of the human growth hormone response to a 6 s and a 30 s cycle ergnometer." *Journal of Sports Sciences* 20 (2002) 487–494. doi: 10.1080/02640410252925152.

Van Cauter, Eve, and Kristen L. Knutson. "Sleep and the Epidemic of Obesity in Children and Adults." *European Journal of Endocrinology* 159 (2008): 559–566. doi:10.1530/EJE-08-0298.

Vicennati, Valentina, Francesca Pasqui, Carla Cavazza, and Renato Pasquali. "Stress-Related Development of Obesity and Cortisol in Women." *Obesity* 17 (2009): 1678–1683. doi:10.1038/oby.2009.76.

Wahl, Patrick. "Hormonal and Metabolic Responses to High Intensity Interval Training." *Sports Medicine and Doping Studies* 3 (2013): 1–2. doi:0.4172/2161-0673.1000e132.

Chapter Seventeen: Don't Forget About Supplements

Aasheim, Erlend T., et al. "Vitamin B Status in Morbidly Obese Patients: A Cross-Sectional Study." *American Journal of Clinical Nutrition* 91 (2008): 362–369. ajcn.nutrition.org/content/87/2/362.long.

Anton, Stephen D., et al. "Effects of Chromium Picolinate on Food Intake and Satiety." *Diabetes Technology & Therapeutics* 10 (2008): 405–412. doi:10.1089/dia.2007.0292.

Bastin, Jean, Alexandra Lopes-Costa, and Fatima Djouadi. "Exposure to Resveratrol Triggers Pharmacological Correction of Fatty Acid Utilization in Human Fatty Acid Oxidation-Deficient Fibroblasts." *Human Molecular Genetics* 20 (2011): 2048–2057. doi:10.1093/hmg/ddr089.

Beezhold, Bonnie, Carol S. Johnston, and Pamela D. Swan. "Vitamin C Depletion Reduces Fat Oxidation at Rest in Obese Adults Consuming a Calorie-Restricted Diet." *Journal of the Federation of American Societies for Experimental Biology* 20 (2006): A608.

Brand-Miller, J. C., et al. "Effects of PGX, a Novel Functional Fibre, on Acute and Delayed Post-prandial Glycaemia." *European Journal of Clinical Nutrition* 64 (2010): 1488–1493. doi:10.1038/ejcn.2010.199.

Castro, Maria C., et al. "Lipoic Acid Prevents Liver Metabolic Changes Induced by Administration of a Fructose-Rich Diet." *Biochimica et Biophysica Acta (BBA)* 1830 (2013): 2226–2232. doi: 10.1016/j.bbagen.2012.10.010.

Chen, Yu-Kuo, et al. "Effects of Green Tea Polyphenol ({dec45})-Epigallocatechin-3-gallate on Newly Developed High-Fat/Western-Style Diet-Induced Obesity and Metabolic Syndrome in Mice." *Journal of Agricultural and Food Chemistry* 59 (2011): 11862–11871. doi:10.1021/jf2029016.

Cheng, Hoi Lun, et al. "Impact of Diet and Weight Loss on Iron and Zinc Status in Overweight and Obese Young Women." *Asia Pacific Journal of Clinical Nutrition* 22 (2013): 574–582. doi:10.6133/apjcn.2013.22.4.08.

Chiang, En-Pei, et al. "Inflammation Causes Tissue-Specific Depletion of Vitamin B6." *Arthritis Research & Therapy* 7 (2005): R1254–R1262. doi:10.1186/ar1821.

Choi, Hye Duck, et al. "Effects of Astaxanthin on Oxidative Stress in Overweight and Obese Adults." *Phytotherapy Research* 25 (2011): 1813–1818. doi:10.1002/ptr.3494.

Ejaz, Asma, Dayong Wu, Paul Kwan, and Mohsen Meydani. "Curcumin Inhibits Adipogenesis in 3T3-L1 Adipocytes and Angiogenesis and Obesity in C57/BL Mice." *Journal of Nutrition* 139 (2009): 919–925. doi:10.3945/jn.108.100966.

Frisco, Simonetta, et al. "Low Circulating Vitamin B_6 Is Associated with Elevation of the Inflammation Marker C-Reactive Protein Independently of Plasma Homocysteine Levels." *Circulation* 103 (2001): 2788–2791. doi: 10.1161/01.CIR.103.23.2788.

Ghanim, Husam, et al. "A Resveratrol and Polyphenol Preparation Suppresses Oxidative and Inflammatory Stress Response to a High-Fat, High-Carbohydrate Meal." *Journal of Clinical Endocrinology and Metabolism* 96 (2011): 1409–1414. doi:10.1210/jc.2010-1812.

Hill, Alison M., Jonathan D. Buckley, Karen J. Murphy, and Peter R. C. Howe. "Combining Fish-Oil Supplements with Regular Aerobic Exercise Improves Body Composition and Cardiovascular

Disease Risk Factors." *American Journal of Clinical Nutrition* 85 (2007): 1267–1274. ajcn.nutrition. org/content/85/5/1267.long.

Ikeuchi, Mayumi, Tomoyuki Koyama, Jiro Takahashi, and Kazunaga Yazawa. "Effects of Astaxanthin in Obese Mice Fed a High-Fat Diet." *Bioscience, Biotechnology, and Biochemistry* 71 (2007): 893–899. doi:10.1271/bbb.60521.

Johnston, Carol S. "Strategies for Healthy Weight Loss: From Vitamin C to the Glycemic Response." *Journal of the American College of Nutrition* 24 (2005): 158–165.

Johnston, Carol S., Bonnie L. Beezhold, Bo Mostow, and Pamela D. Swan. "Plasma Vitamin C Is Inversely Related to Body Mass Index and Waist Circumference but Not to Plasma Adiponectin in Nonsmoking Adults." *Journal of Nutrition* 137 (2007): 1757–1762. jn.nutrition.org/content/137/7/1757.long.

Kaats, Gilbert R., Kenneth Blum, Jeffrey A. Fisher, and Jack A. Adelman. "Effects of Chromium Picolinate Supplementation on Body Composition: A Randomized, Double-Masked, Placebo-Controlled Study." *Current Therapeutic Research* 57 (1996): 747–756. doi:10.1016/S0011-393X(96)80080-4.

Kinscherf, R., et al. "Low Plasma Glutamine in Combination with High Glutamate Levels Indicate Risk for Loss of Body Cell Mass in Healthy Individuals: The Effect of N-Acetyl-Cysteine." *Journal of Molecular Medicine* 74 (1996): 393–400. doi:10.1007/BF00210633.

LeBlanc, Erin S., et al. "Associations Between 25-Hydroxyvitamin D and Weight Gain in Elderly Women." *Journal of Women's Health* 21 (2012): 1066–1073. doi:10.1089/jwh.2012.3506.

Lee, Bor-Jen, Yi-Chai Huang, Shu-Ju Chen, and Ping-Ting Lin. "Effects of Coenzyme Q10 Supplementation on Inflammatory Markers (High-Sensitivity C-Reactive Protein, Interleukin-6, and Homocysteine) in Patients with Coronary Artery Disease." *Nutrition* 28 (2012): 767–772. doi:10.1016/j.nut.2011.11.008.

Liel, Y. "Low Circulating Vitamin D in Obesity." *Calcified Tissue International* 43 (1988): 199–210. http://www.ncbi.nlm.nih.gov/pubmed/3145124

Lyon, Michael R., and Ronald G. Reichert. "The Effect of a Novel Viscous Polysaccharide Along with Lifestyle Changes on Short-Term Weight Loss and Associated Risk Factors in Overweight and Obese Adults: An Observational Retrospective Clinical Program Analysis." *Alternative Medicine Review* 15 (2010): 68–75. www.altmedrev.com/publications/15/1/68.pdf.

Machado, Susan. "Nutrient 'Cocktail' Delays Aging and Extends Life Span." *Life Extension Magazine* (2012). www.lef.org/magazine/mag2012/may2012_Nutrient-Cocktail-Delays-Aging-Extends-Life-Span_01.htm.

Noland, Robert C., et al. "Carnitine Insufficiency Caused by Aging and Overnutrition Compromises Mitochondrial Performance and Metabolic Control." *Journal of Biological Chemistry* 284 (2009): 22840–22852. doi:10.1074/jbc.M109.032888.

Noreen, Eric E., et al., "Effects of Supplemental Fish Oil on Resting Metabolic Rate, Body Composition, and Salivary Cortisol in Healthy Adults." *Journal of the International Society of Sports Nutrition* 7 (2010): 1–7. doi:10.1186/1550-2783-7-31.

Packer, Lester, Eric H. Witt, and Hans Jügen Tritschler.. "Alpha-Lipoic Acid as a Biological Antioxidant." *Free Radical Biology and Medicine* 19 (1995): 227–250. doi:10.1016/0891-5849(95)00017-R.

Reimer, R. A., et al. "Increased Plasma PYY Levels Following Supplementation with the Functional Fiber PolyGlycopleX in Healthy Adults." *European Journal of Clinical Nutrition* 64 (2010): 1186–1191. doi:10.1038/ejcn.2010.141.

Richards, J. Brent. "Higher Serum Vitamin D Concentrations Are Associated with Longer Leukocyte Telomere Length in Women." *American Journal of Clinical Nutrition* 86 (2007): 1420–1425. ajcn.nutrition.org/content/86/5/1420.long.

Rosenblum, Jennifer L., Victor M. Castro, Carolyn E. Moore, and Lee M. Kaplan. "Calcium and Vitamin D Supplementation Is Associated with Decreased Abdominal Visceral Adipose Tissue in Overweight and Obese Adults." *American Journal of Clinical Nutrition* (2012). doi:0.3945/ajcn.111.019489.

Santos-González, Mónica, Consuelo Gómez Díaz, Plácido Navas, and José Manuel Villalba. "Modifications of Plasma Proteome in Long-Lived Rats Fed on a Coenzyme Q10-Supplemented Diet." *Experimental Gerontology* 42 (2007): 798–806. doi:10.1016/j.exger.2007.04.013.

Senger, A. E. Vieira, C. H. A. Schwanke, I. Gomes, and Maria Gabriela Valle Gottlieb. "Effect of Green Tea (*Camellia sinensis*) Consumption on the Components of Metabolic Syndrome in Elderly." *Journal of Nutrition, Health and Aging* 16 (2012): 738–742. doi:10.1007/s12603-012-0081-5.

Shehzad, Adeeb, Taewook Ha, Fazli Subhan, and Young Sup Lee. "New Mechanisms and the Anti-inflammatory Role of Curcumin in Obesity and Obesity-Related Metabolic Diseases." *European Journal of Nutrition* 50 (2011): 151–161. doi:10.1007/s00394-011-0188-1.

Shen, Jian, et al. "Association of Vitamin B-6 Status with Inflammation, Oxidative Stress, and Chronic Inflammatory Conditions: The Boston Puerto Rican Health Study." *American Journal of Clinical Nutrition* 91 (2010): 337–342. doi: 10.3945/ajcn.2009.28571.

Tsuge, H., N. Hotta, and T Hayakawa. "Effects of Vitamin B-6 on (n–3) Polyunsaturated Fatty Acid Metabolism." *Journal of Nutrition* 130 (2000): 333S–334S. jn.nutrition.org/content/130/2/333.long.

Valdecantos, M. Pillar, et al. "Lipoic Acid Administration Prevents Nonalcoholic Steatosis Linked to Long-Term High-Fat Feeding by Modulating Mitochondrial Function." *Journal of Nutritional Biochemistry* 23 (2012): 1676–1684. doi: 10.1016/j.jnutbio.2011.11.011.

Vincent, John B. "Chromium—The Potential Value and Toxicity of Chromium Picolinate as a Nutritional Supplement, Weight Loss Agent and Muscle Development Agent." *Sports Medicine* 33 (2003): 213–230. doi:10.2165/00007256-200333030-00004.

Xu, Qun, et al. "Multivitamin Use and Telomere Length in Women." *American Journal of Clinical Nutrition* 89 (2009): 1857–1863. doi:10.3945/ajcn.2008.26986.

Yubero-Serrano, Elena M., et al. "Mediterranean Diet Supplemented with Coenzyme Q10 Modifies the Expression of Proinflammatory and Endoplasmic Reticulum Stress-Related Genes in Elderly Men and Women." *Journals of Gerontology. Series A, Biological Sciences & Medical Sciences* 67 (2012): 3–10. doi:10.1093/gerona/glr167.

Yun, Jung-Mi, Alexander Chien, Ishwarlal Jialal, and Sridevi Devaraj. "Resveratrol Upregulates SIRT1 and Inhibits Cellular Oxidative Stress in the Diabetic Milieu: Mechanistic Insights." *Journal of Nutritional Biochemistry* 23 (2012): 699–705.

Zhao, W., et al. "Protective Effects of Astaxanthin Against Oxidative Damage Induced By 60Co Gamma-Ray Irradiation." *Journal of Hygiene Research* 40 (2011): 551–554. europepmc.org/abstract/MED/22043699/.

INDEX